COMPUTERS IN HUMAN SERVICES

COMPUTERS IN HUMAN SERVICES
An Overview for Clinical and Welfare Services

Edited by

John T. Pardeck
Southeast Missouri State University,
Cape Girardeau, USA

and

John W. Murphy
University of Miami,
Florida, USA

harwood academic publishers
chur • london • paris • new york • melbourne

Harwood Academic Publishers

Post Office Box 197
London WC2E 9PX
United Kingdom

58, rue Lhomond
75005 Paris
France

Post Office Box 786
Cooper Station
New York, New York 10276
United States of America

Private Bag 8
Camberwell, Victoria 3124
Australia

Library of Congress Cataloging-in-Publication Data

Computers in human services.

1. Medical informatics. 2. Medicine--Data processing.
3. Social services--Data processing. I. Pardeck, John T.
II. Murphy, John W. [DNLM: 1. Computers. 2. Medical
Informatics. 3. Social Work. W 26.5 C74575]
R858.C6543 1989 610'.285 89-26685
ISBN 3-7186-5009-6
ISBN 3-7186-5005-3 (pbk.)

Printed in the United Kingdom by Bell & Bain Ltd., Glasgow.

Contents

About the Editors

John W. Murphy is Associate Professor of Sociology in the Department of Sociology, University of Miami. He received his Ph.D. degree from Ohio State University, and has worked in both applied and academic settings. In addition to books and articles related to social philosophy and methodology, he has edited the *Underside of High Tech* and *Technology and Human Productivity* (with John T. Pardeck). Dr. Murphy is the author of numerous articles on computer technology and social service delivery.

John T. Pardeck is currently Professor of Social Work and Chairperson of the Department of Social Work at Southeast Missouri State University. He was formerly Director of the Social Work Program at Arkansas State University and a Researcher for the Region VI Child Welfare Training Center, Tulane University School of Social Work. His research interests include child welfare, computers, and issues related to child and family development. Dr. Pardeck is the author of *The Forgotten Children: A Study of the Stability and Continuity of Foster Care* and co-author of *Child Welfare Training and Practice*, *Young People with Problems: A Guide to Bibliotherapy*, *Books for Early Childhood: A Developmental Perspective*, and *Technology and Human Productivity: Challenges for the Future*. He has published articles in such journals as *Social Work*, *International Journal of Social Psychiatry*, *International Social Work*, *Child Abuse and Neglect*, *Personality and Individual Differences*, and *Group Psychotherapy, Psychodrama, and Sociometry*. Dr. Pardeck is Associate Editor of the *Journal of Sociology and Social Welfare* and is on the editorial board of *Early Child Development and Care* and *Family Therapy*. He is a member of the Academy of Certified Social Workers and is a Licensed Certified Social Worker. Dr. Pardeck was elected to Phi Kappa Phi academic honor society in 1974 and received his M.S.W. and Ph.D. in social work from the School of Social Service, Saint Louis University.

About the Contributors

Karen A. Callaghan received her Ph.D. degree from Ohio State University. Currently, she is Adjunct Associate Professor of Sociology at the University of Miami, Coral Gables, FL. She has worked for years in the field of mental health and child welfare, and has published various articles related to the delivery of social services.

Ruby C. Chittenden received her B.S. degree in Business Education from Morehead State University and M.A. in Business from Western Kentucky University. She is a faculty member at Arkansas State University in the Computer Information Systems Department.

Harold P. Erdman received his Ph.D. in Industrial Engineering from the University of Wisconsin-Madison. He is currently Lead Systems Analyst at Health Care 2000, in San Francisco, CA. His area of interest is computer applications to health care, including computer-based assessment, expert systems and patient education. His most recent publications include "A computer consultation system for primary care physicians" and "Direct patient-computer interviewing."

Sharon W. Foster received her Ph.D. in Clinical Psychology from the University of Illinois at Urbana-Champaign. She is currently a Clinical Instructor in the Department of Pediatrics at the University of Wisconsin-Madison, where she is a staff psychologist in the General Pediatric and Teenage Clinic. Her interests include the study of family interaction and patient adherence to medical regimens.

Dr. Terry Holbrook is Director of Social Work at Willard Psychiatric Center in Willard, N.Y. He has an M.S.W. from the State University at Albany, N.Y. and a Ph.D. in Social Work from The Union of Experimenting Colleges and Universities, Cincinnati, Ohio. His most recent publication entitled "Policing Sexuality in a Modern State Hospital" was published in *Hospital and Community Psychiatry* in January, 1989. His interests include organizational influences upon professional behavior, quality assurance, and case records. Address correspondence to 4056 Allens Hill Rd., Holcomb, N.Y. 14469.

Dr. Howard Jacob Karger is Associate Professor and Director of Doctoral Education, School of Social Work, Louisiana State University. He has written in the area of administration and is the author of *The Sentinels of Order* (Lanham, MD: University Press of America, 1987); *Social Workers and Labor Unions* (New York: Greenwood Press, 1988); and with David Stoesz, *American Social Welfare Policy* (New York: Longman, 1989).

Dr. Michael J. Kelly is Associate Professor, School of Social Work, University of Missouri-Columbia. He has written in the area of administration and continuing education in social work.

Larry W. Kreuger is Assistant Professor, School of Social Work, University of Missouri-Columbia where he teaches research and social policy courses in the graduate social work program. He has designed several computerized data bases used for evaluation of delivery of services to homeless populations in St. Louis. He has published articles on computer applications in *Social Work, Computers in Human Services, Early Child Development and Care, Journal of Independent Social Work*, and *Journal of Compliance in Health Care.*

John W. Murphy is Associate Professor of Sociology at the University of Miami, Coral Gables, FL. He received his Ph.D. degree from Ohio State University. His interests include social theory, program evaluation, and the study of technology. He has published numerous articles in a variety of areas. His most recent books include *The Underside of High-tech, Technology and Human Productivity* (with J.T. Pardeck), and *Postmodern Social Analysis and Criticism.*

John T. Pardeck, Ph.D., is Professor of Social Work and Chair of the Department of Social Work at Southeast Missouri State University. His most recent publications include *Technology and Human Productivity, Books for Early Childhood: A Developmental Perspective*, and *Microcomputers in Early Childhood Education.* He is also the author of numerous articles on computers and therapeutic intervention.

Joseph J. Pilotta, Ph.D., is Associate Professor of Communication at Ohio State University. He received doctorates from Ohio University and the University of Toronto. His most recent books are *Responsive Institutions: A Communication Order Without Control* and *Qualitative Methodology, Theory and Application: A Guide for the Social Practitioner* (with John W. Murphy).

John J. Stretch is Professor and Director of the Doctoral Program, School of Social Service, Saint Louis University, where he teaches policy, evaluation research, and programming, planning, and budgeting in the graduate and doctoral programs. He has directed numerous evaluation projects involving the application of technology to solve human services management problems. He has published in *Social Work, Administration in Social Work, Community Mental Health Journal, Child Welfare, Social Casework*, and other journals.

Dr. John S. Wodarski is currently the Associate Vice President of Research and Graduate Studies at The University of Akron, Akron, Ohio. He was the Director of the Research Center at the University of Georgia from 1978-1988. He has had substantial interest in computers throughout his career. Dr. Wodarski is the author of over 300 published papers and 15 texts. His major area of interest includes child abuse, family violence, adolescent substance abuse and the use of computers in behavioral science.

1

Introduction

John W. Murphy, PhD
Associate Professor of Sociology, Department of Sociology, University of Miami

John T. Pardeck, MSW, PhD
Professor and Chair, Department of Social Work, Southeast Missouri State University

Technology is currently proliferating throughout society at an unprecedented rate. For example, computers can be found in homes, schools, and factories. Social service agencies are no exception to this trend. Computer programs are available that can conduct in-take interviews, monitor treatment plans, administer and score clinical instruments, and even engage clients in therapeutic dialogue. Indeed, some critics claim that service delivery has come to be mediated completely by technology (Murphy and Pardeck, 1986a).

Most germane to this discovery is that computers are not simply tools. While using unique imagery, Berdyaev (1963) writes that technology has "cosmological implications". Although he adopts different language, Jacques Ellul (1964) makes a similar point. He charges that modern society is governed by a "technological ethic". In each case, the idea is that computers "manipulate symbols", rather than merely crunch numbers (Boden, 1977, pp.15-17). In other words, computers create a unique presence in an organization, which requires that life be altered in many significant ways. Some of these changes are merely logistical, while others are conceptual (Murphy, Pardeck, Nolden, and Pilotta, 1987).

As opposed to tools, computers are not passive. Those who plan to purchase and implement computer technology should be aware of this factor. The mere presence of a computer has impact on the physical surroundings within an agency. Work schedules, communication patterns, and job designs may be negatively influenced. Disruption, however, may not be limited to environmental and logistical considerations. If this were the case, the problems brought about by computerization would be relatively easy to solve. But the use of computers has a conceptual "underside" that usually goes unnoticed, until difficulties arise. In short, computers are accompanied by what some authors call a "world-view", which embodies assumptions that must be accepted as valid if these devices are to operate effectively (Murphy and

Pardeck, 1985). These presuppositions, accordingly, require that reality be construed in a way that may undermine the delivery of social services.

According to Ellul (1964) and Winner (1977), modern societies have become enslaved to technology. Machines that were supposed to conserve labor energy, have not increased leisure time. All that has happened is a plethora of technical problems must be corrected, within the confines of the traditional workday. Additionally, a new level of bureaucracy has been created, in order to handle technical issues. On the more conceptual side, workers seem to have become dominated by their own creations. The pace of a job, the type of data that can be collected, and even the questions that can be raised, appear to be dictated by what is believed to be technically feasible. Through computerization time, space, and cognition are given a technical cast, which eventually may become very problematic.

Before computer technology will enhance the delivery of social services, practitioners must expand their view of technology. They must remember one theme: the thrust of technology is not necessarily technical. Stated differently, without an accompanying culture of technology, computers would be useless. Central to this culture is a willingness to give primacy to technological rationality, as opposed to other styles of reasoning. Coincident with this demarche, the physical and conceptual changes mandated by computerization are readily accepted.

Associated with technological rationality is the belief that objective knowledge exists, and, accordingly, this information can be obtained through improved methodological rigor. In other words, at the basis of technological rationality is dualism, which supports differentiating the world into two opposing parts. Traditionally these factors have been referred to as subjectivity and objectivity. Once this bifurcation is accepted, however, the human element - or interpretation - is identified as a prime source of opinion or error. What this means is that practically any maneuver is justified, in order to suppress interpretation. After all, the discovery of truth hangs in the balance.

As a result of this desire to control interpretation, commentators have begun to argue that social life is now regulated by a "technological imperative" (Davis, 1986). At every opportunity, therefore, technological devices should be incorporated into a task. The rationale for this action is quite simple: technology is thought to be undaunted by situational exigencies, and thus any job that is computerized will likely be undertaken with precision. With subjectivity moved to the periphery of the workplace, the argument is that productivity and efficiency can only improve. The same logic is applied to the delivery of social services. A computerized diagnosis, for example, will probably be more comprehensive and accurate than one rendered by a therapist (Kleinmuntz, 1984).

No-one should be surprised, accordingly, when the social side of computer use is ignored. If human judgments can be translated into technical operations, writes Lewis Mumford (1963), objectivity and precision are thought to be enhanced. In point of fact, emotional control has been cited as the motive that sustains the implementation of technology (Berger, Berger, and Kellner, 1973). By design the human element is obscured. Planners who are enamored of technological rationality have no compunction about dehumanizing a procedure, even those essential to the delivery of human services.

In this book, technology is treated as more than a tool. Along with logistical concerns, research, moral-ethical, philosophical, and organizational issues are discussed. Implicit is that a favorable human dimension must be engendered, or computer technology will not facilitate the work done by therapists and other health care professionals. This contention is unique among practitioners, for recent research suggests that they view computers to consist of little more than hardware and software (Pardeck, Collier, and Murphy, 1987). If the most sophisticated technology is purchased, the belief is that service delivery will be upgraded. Nonetheless, this optimism is not warranted, according to computer theorists. Various experts in the area of artificial intelligence, for instance, suggest that unless key aspects of human cognition are built into computer programs, decision making will not become more reliable because of computerization. Correspondingly, social factors must not be diminished in importance when formulating the plans for a computer system. Without a congenial human-machine interface, the utility of computer technology will undoubtedly decrease. This quite controversial statement should be remembered by social practitioners, when they are preparing their agencies to enter the so-called computer age.

LOGISTICAL ISSUES

Usually practitioners are concerned with the type of equipment that will be installed. Hence software and hardware are their focus of attention. For example, discussions are devoted to the amount of memory space required to complete a job, in addition to the number of work stations that will be needed. Further, a computer must be powerful enough to perform the analyses that are desired.

Yet even at the technical end of computer use, other than technological concerns must be addressed. The flow of information must be charted, so that data move effectively throughout an organization. Even the best computer is useless, if the source, path, and destination of information are not identified. Also, workers must be able to learn rapidly how to use a computer. Therefore, models should be selected with respect to the personnel pattern present in an agency. The conditions under which a computer will be used are also important. For example, the admissions office in a community mental health center is often chaotic, and thus a very complicated device will not likely simplify the in-take process. Patient data, additionally, must be kept confidential. Policies and procedures must be established to determine who will have access to a client's file.

Though these are logistical concerns, technological solutions alone are insufficient. Certainly a systems analyst can pinpoint appropriate locations for data entry that are cost-effective. Nonetheless, unless these technical experts are familiar with the intricacies of the agencies they are analyzing, efficient but irrelevant computer packages may be adopted. In short, technical expertise is no substitute for human relations. Japanese managers have recognized this point, and contend that the proper "cultural software" is crucial to the success of a computer system (Pardeck and Murphy, 1986). Without a policy pertaining to a back-up strategy, for example, data may not be preserved during a power failure. Guaranteeing the safety and utility of information is not simply a technological problem.

TECHNOLOGY AS PHILOSOPHY

Recognized by many writers is that computers operate on the basis of a "micro-world" (Murphy and Pardeck, 1986b). Particular philosophical principles, in other words, are vital to the operation of a computer. Because data processing consists of "reading" input, information must be conceptualized in a special manner. Writers such as Lyotard (1984) Baudrillard (1983) and the Dreyfuses (1986) maintain that the information "bit" is the form of knowledge most compatible with computerization. Knowledge assumes this identity following the acceptance of three rules. First, data are material objects. Second, mathematics is most appropriate for labelling these entities. And third, the logic of data classification reflects reality. Data are deanimated successfully due to these assumptions, which are the centerpiece of the computer micro-world.

Because data that are ambiguous cannot be easily processed, the element of interpretation must be removed from the activity whereby data are categorized. Therefore, input can be adjusted neatly to its "address space" (Bolter, 1984, pp. 83-90). Yet understanding data to be concatenated pieces of knowledge can have dire consequences. Indeed, language comes to be viewed as an inanimate system, which can be dissected and analyzed in an almost unlimited variety of ways. Lost, however, is the expressiveness indigenous to speech. The situational relevance of facts is also minimized, because valid knowledge is equated with empirical indicators. But can an accurate diagnosis, for example, be based on knowledge that is purged of interpretation and human passion? Many therapists believe that unless a client's understanding of reality is appreciated, intervention will be, at best, haphazard. They argue that judgments determine whether or not a particular behavior is treated as indicative of mental illness. Insight must be gained into these interpretive acts, accordingly, before a relevant course of therapy can be prescribed.

Practitioners should be aware that computer use is underpinned by a philosophy sometimes referred to as realism. Most important, this viewpoint may begin to influence many aspects of service delivery that are not linked immediately to technical skills. Language, facts, and social problems may be misconstrued as divorced from interpretation and readily classifiable. As a result, the *art* of intervention may atrophy, once a client's self-understanding is deemed to be an impediment to gathering factual clinical data. That is, a therapist's ability to search for and decipher evidence may deteriorate. Practitioners must not allow their vision to be narrowed by the computer micro-world, so that knowledge becomes one-dimensional. For when the amount of information about a client's condition is unduly truncated, the delivery of social services suffers.

MORAL DILEMMAS

Due to the emphasis placed on quantification by computerization, a variety of moral questions are attendant to computer use. Particularly, computer mediated intervention has been called dehumanizing. Due to the value attributed to standardization and objectivity, computerized assessments have a tendency to become synonymous with testing (Matarazzo, 1986). The administration, scoring, and interpretation of computerized clinical instruments is extremely formalized, thereby reducing to a minimum human error. No wonder this method of clinical evaluation is attractive. But do tests reveal a comprehensive picture of a client? Opponents of computerized therapy say no. In fact, they charge that the significance of data is derived from the framework or context within which this information resides. A client's social environment, not to mention emotional factors, cannot be easily conceptualized, in the rigid manner required for data processing. Therefore, qualitative features of social existence are ignored, while clients are insensitively treated. Long-term, in-depth treatment may be avoided or replaced by more ephemeral remedies. To some therapists, such standardization is tantamount to manipulation.

Another undesirable consequence of the ease with which computerized instruments are administered, is that "quick and dirty" assessments may become all too common. In the hands of technical experts, intervention may become nothing more than a surreptitious means of social control. The owners of a factory, for example, may employ a testing service to monitor workers. Also, school officials and police officers may get into the testing business, because the requisite technical skills are so easy to acquire. The aim of evaluation in these instances may be to eliminate troublemakers, rather than to solve problems.

A third general area of concern relates to the possibility of computers further increasing the power of therapists. Most persons are intimidated by the prospect of seeking professional help (Murphy and Pardeck, 1986c). How are their fears to be calmed if a computer is interjected into the client-therapist relationship? Because a computer may be seen as supplying a practitioner with an unimpeachable "second opinion", clients may be reluctant to challenge a diagnosis. The idea that therapists are infallible scientists may only be encouraged, thereby reinforcing the asymmetry that often exists between practitioners and their clients.

In terms of creating moral dilemmas, computers are not neutral. A situation may be generated through their use where clients are misinterpreted, intimidated, or, possibly, manipulated. Most practitioners strive to avoid this sort of misconduct. Doubtless, bias and coercion are supposed to be passé, as a result of computerization. Yet practitioners should not be so naive as to think that immoral or unprofessional behavior cannot be instigated by a computer.

ORGANIZATIONAL STRATEGIES

As part of establishing a milieu for effective computer use, a variety of organizational development strategies may be helpful. When organized as a bureaucracy, an agency is fragmented. Computerization may only aggravate this situation. Each department may establish a separate data base, generate different reports, and hoard information. Giving various segments of an organization direct access to data may inaugurate internecine competition, which may prove to be very costly. As a substitute for bureaucracy, for example, a "linking-pin" style of organization can increase the usefulness of computers (Murphy and Pardeck, 1986d). Developed by Rensis Likert, a key person from each department works temporarily in a number of other units, thereby directly linking components of an organization that were formerly obliquely related. In this way, the information and skills required for computerization to succeed are disseminated smoothly throughout an agency.

As should be noted, computerization represents change. Researchers have known for some time that a particular style of management assists workers to cope with adjustments in their daily routines. Specifically, practitioners must be encouraged to participate, as early as possible, in planning sessions. Workers tend to resist change less when they are fully informed about coming events. Many businesses are discovering that the formation of "key report" groups can be very beneficial, with respect to coordinating the implementation and use of computers (Namm, 1986). Strategic employees are assembled to examine the data needs of an organization, such as the purpose for gathering information, the amount of data to be collected, and the types of reports to be generated. Additionally, the training and other support workers needs can be outlined. The fears workers may have about computers can be significantly alleviated, if the plans for both change and remediation are openly discussed.

Computers should not be viewed as merely an adjunct to an organization. As suggested earlier, the structure of an agency may be affected adversely by computers. On the other hand, management practices can be instituted that have proven to be effective in reducing the problems often associated with organizational change. Practitioners should be cognizant of these methods.

CONCLUSION

Although computerization is supposed to create an aura of objectivity, practitioners should not be blinded by this illusion. Actually, a unique context of interaction, the validity of particular values, and special social imagery are presupposed by the operation of computers. In other words, these devices lend legitimacy to a specific, and quite esoteric, portrayal of reality. Practitioners, therefore, must begin to imagine how they can be unwittingly manipulated by computers. Critics of computerized intervention suggest that if practitioners are not vigilant, computer technology may undermine the person-in-environment approach to service delivery. Yet this *modus operandi* has been identified as basic to socially sensitive treatment (Stewart, 1988). Due to the pre-eminence of the computer micro-world and the information "bit", holistic analysis is not necessarily a strength of computerization.

In this book the attempt is made to approach holistically the application of computers to the delivery of social services. Technical concerns are not the center of attention, however they are not overlooked. When logistical issues are examined, they are placed in a human context. The hope is that readers will be given a broader view of computerization than is typically the case. As a result, maybe computers will enhance, rather than detract from service delivery.

REFERENCES

Baudrillard, J. (1983). *In the Shadow of the Silent Majorities*. New York: Semiotext (e).

Berdyaev, N. (1963). *The Fate of Man in the Modern World*. Ann Arbor: The University of Michigan Press.

Boden, M. (1977). *Artificial Intelligence and Natural Man*. New York: Basic Books.

Bolter, J. D. (1984). *Turing's Man: Western Culture in the Computer Age*. Chapel Hill: University of North Carolina Press.

Davis, D. D. (1986). *Managing Technological Innovation*. San Francisco: Jossey-Bass.

Dreyfus, H. L. and Dreyfus, S. E. (1986). *Mind over Machine*. New York: The Free Press.

Ellul, J. (1984). *The Technological Society*. New York: Random House.

Kleinmuntz, B. (1984). "The Scientific Study of Clinical Judgment in Psychology and Medicine". *Clinical Psychology Review*, 4, 111-126.

Lyotard, J. F. (1984). *The Postmodern Condition: A Report on Knowledge*. Minneapolis: University of Minnesota Press.

Matarazzo, J. D. (1986). "Computerized Clinical Test Interpretations: Unvalidated Plus All Mean and No Sigma: *American Psychologist*, 41, 14-24.

Mumford, L. (1963). *Technics and Civilization.* New York: Harcourt, Brace, and World.

Murphy, J. W., and Pardeck, J. T. (1986a). "Technologically Mediated Therapy: A Critique". *Social Casework*, 67, 605-612.

Murphy, J. W. and Pardeck, J. T. (1986b). "Computers and Cognitive Development: A Preliminary Statement". *Early Childhood Development and Care* 25, 221-230.

Murphy, J. W. and Pardeck, J. T. (1986c). "Technology and the Manufacture of Madness: A New Dimension". *International Journal of Social Psychiatry*, 32, 41-46.

Murphy, J. W. and Pardeck, J. T. (1986d). "The 'Burnout Syndrome' and Management Style". *The Clinical Supervisor*, 4, 35-44.

Murphy, J. W., Pardeck, J. T., Nolden, W., and Pilotta, J. J. (1987). "Conceptual Issues Related to the Use of Computers in Social Work Practice: *Journal of Independent Social Work*, 1, 63-73.

Namm, D. (1986). "The Case of the Changing Technology: Impact of Micro-Computer Technology in a *Fortune* 500 Company. In J. W. Murphy and J. T. Pardeck (Eds.), *Technology and Human Productivity* (pp.95-101). Westport, CT: Greenwood Press.

Pardeck, J. T. Collier, K. and Murphy, J. W. (1987) "The Use and Perception of Computers by Professional Social Workers". *Family Therapy*, 14, 1-8.

Stewart, R. (1988). "Social Work Practice in a High-tech Era". In J. W. Murphy and J. T. Pardeck (Eds)., *Technology and Human Service Delivery: Challenges and a Critical Perspective.* New York: Haworth.

Winner, L. (1977). *Autonomous Technology: Technics-out-of-control as a Theme in Political Thought.* Cambridge, MA: MIT Press.

2

Computer Information Systems

Ruby Chittenden
College of Business, Arkansas State University

The change from a manual information system to a computer information system requires an investment in time and money. While the money aspect may not be surprising, both managers and workers should be aware that a significant amount of time is needed to learn how to operate a computerized information system. Implementing this sort of system, in short, involves much more than just purchasing a computer. While a computer is necessary, knowing which brand and size of computer to buy presents tremendous problems to the novice.

There are five aspects to a computer system: hardware, software, data, procedures, and personnel. To have an efficient computer system, no aspect should be neglected.It is also critical to understand security problems and the procedures for developing a new computer system, including non-technological issues.

HARDWARE

There are three basic sizes of computers today: microcomputers, minicomputers, and main frame computers. The differences in these computers include memory size, speed, and number of peripheral devices they will accept.

Memory size is very important. Every computer has a Central Processing Unit (CPU) which includes an arithmetic/logic unit, a control unit, and main memory. Before data processing can begin, information must be placed in the main memory of the CPU. Of course, a large enough memory must be available to hold a program and all of the necessary data.

A very important concept to understand is that data is stored inside the CPU as magnetized areas. The smallest magnetized area is called a BIT; the bit can be turned on or turned off (actually, magnetized in one direction or the opposite). Since a bit is too small to store a letter of the alphabet or a number, bits are grouped together into BYTEs. In most computers a byte contains eight bits, and a code called the Extended Binary Coded Decimal Interchange Code (EBCDIC) has been devised to represent letters of the alphabet, numbers, and symbols.

It is important to understand that when data are read from an input device or typed in from a computer keyboard, each piece of information must be recorded in the main memory of the CPU before any processing can take place. Once the data are placed in the main memory under the control of a computer program they can be processed to produce the required output.

Now, back to memory size. Today, computers can be purchased with as many as 16 million bytes of storage. Memory size, however, is described in terms of "K". "K" represents approximately one thousand bytes of storage. "M" refers to megabytes, or a million bytes of storage. So, when a computer is advertised as having 64 K, this means it has 64,000 bytes of storage in the main memory of the CPU. In other words, this particular model can store 64,000 letters of the alphabet, numbers, or symbols.

Why is this important? If a computer is to be used to keep track of inventory or to produce payroll information, all the necessary data and the inventory program must be able to reside in the main memory of the computer. If the memory is too small, a program may not be able to be processed. So, the size of a computer depends upon the amount of data that will be used.

One of the first questions a computer salesperson will ask is: "How much memory do you need?" Before entering a computer store, a good deal of time should be spent researching the types and sizes of computers that are available. There is nothing a computer salesperson loves more than a customer who really does not know what he or she wants, other than a computer. Therefore, the type of work to be done and the amount of data to be processed should be known before purchasing a computer.

Another important concept for the computer novice is that there are two types of computer storage: main memory (inside the CPU) which was just discussed, and secondary storage (permanent storage). Secondary storage allows data to be kept permanently on a secondary storage device. The two most common storage devices are magnetic tape and magnetic disk. Of these two, the magnetic disk is the most popular.

For example, if a computer is used to compute a monthly payroll, all necessary information about the employees will have to be entered into the memory of the CPU. Specifically social security numbers, pay rates, hours worked, deductions, etc. will have to be included. After this data has been introduced, the program will be entered and the data processed according to the instructions in the program. The program will likely produce a payroll report, pay checks, and any other desired output. Much of the data entered during one month will have to be entered again in following months when payroll is again processed. Accordingly, to keep from typing this information each month on the keyboard, that data can be copied from the CPU memory to a magnetic disk where it can be permanently stored.

It is important to understand the difference between storage in the main memory of the CPU and secondary storage. They are two very different concepts. It does not matter how much secondary storage is available, the memory must be large enough to hold data and the required program at the same time.

The first computers were large, bulky, slow machines. As time passed, computers became smaller, faster, more powerful, and cheaper. In the early days, the only computer available was the large main frame version. In the early 1970's, the minicomputer was developed by Digital Equipment Corporation. This opened computer use to smaller companies who could not afford the large main frames and a revolution in computer use followed. Today, microcomputers can be purchased. These small computers have caused their own revolution because of their low cost and ease of use.

Peripheral equipment is also necessary to complete the hardware for a computer system. Peripheral equipment includes: disk drives, tape drives, printers, and additional computer terminals. The size of computer dictates how much peripheral equipment is possible. It is not uncommon for a main frame computer to support hundreds of computer terminals, as well as numerous disk drives and tape drives. A microcomputer can support disk drives, tape drives, and printers, but does not support additional computer terminals.

In addition, a business may also require communication equipment, such as devices which connect a computer to various means of communication, which in turn allow computers to be in contact with one another. A telephone modem is one such device which allows persons to connect their computers to telephone communications lines.

There are many publications which supply hardware information. It is difficult to keep up with the everyday changes occurring in this industry. Therefore, customers should become technically educated before buying a computer. Colleagues who have computer systems should be consulted, in order to get their opinions concerning a computer's good and bad points.

Software

Software is defined as the programs which direct the computer to process data. Hardware is tangible; software is intangible. A computer system is only as good as the programs that are available. A program consists of a list of instructions given to the computer, so that specific output can be produced. There are two basic ways to obtain computer software: programs may be written "in-house" by computer programmers or purchased "off-the-shelf" from software manufacturers.

"Off-the-shelf" programs can be obtained fairly easily, because of the growth of the software industry in recent years. The major problem with purchasing these programs is that they often do not perfectly fit the user's requirements. For example, a program to compute a monthly balance sheet would be written in a general fashion so as to fit as many companies as possible. However, "off-the-shelf" programs can be altered to meet a particular organization's needs. These alterations are made by a computer programmer.

A company or agency may be large enough to have on staff a computer programmer. If this is the case, that person will be able to write computer programs to meet exact specifications. This, however, is a very time consuming task because the programmer needs exact requirements before the program can be designed, coded in a programming language, tested, and then implemented. Clearly purchasing computer programs from a software house is often the most effective strategy.

Computer programs are written in various programming languages. Some languages are designed to accommodate mathematics and science problems, while some are intended to be used in business situations. Science languages include FORTRAN and BASIC; business languages include COBOL, RPG, and BASIC. Nonetheless because a different computer program must often be designed to solve different problems, software may end up costing as much or more than the hardware. This fact is seldom stated, but the potential computer user must be aware of this issue.

Data

When data are processed by a computer system, this information must be organized. Usually this structure is expressed in terms of fields, records, and files. A field is defined as one unit of data; for example, a name, a social security number, an address, or an inventory amount would all be examples of fields. Fields are commonly grouped together to form a record, and records are grouped together to form a file.

These data contained in fields, records, and files are usually stored on some form of secondary storage which is machine readable, such as magnetic tape or magnetic disk. When the data are to be used they are read into the CPU's main memory for processing. Data may also be stored in a secondary unit, using the EBCDIC code which was mentioned earlier in this chapter.

Every time a comment is made regarding the ease with which the computer can process data, remember that at some point someone will have to sit at a computer input device and enter the data needed into storage. For example, if a doctor has fifty patients, a file of fifty records will have to be keyed into storage. Each record will have fields of information on each patient. This Patient File may then be used to produce a desired report. It will be the responsibility of management, working with employees, to decide which pieces of data are to be kept in the files.

Data are processed under the control of a computer program. The computer has the capability of three major functions: input/output operations, arithmetic operations, and logic operations. In the input/output operations, data are recorded on an input device (computer terminal, key-to-disk, or key-to-tape), and then read into the main memory of the computer. Accordingly, the results of that processing are produced as output through an output device (computer terminal screen or printer).

Once data have been stored in main memory, they can be used in addition, subtraction, multiplication, division, and other operations. The results of these operations can be stored in the memory and used in further calculations.

One of the great powers of the computer lies in its ability to make comparisons between numbers, alphabetical characters, or special characters, and to perform other actions based on these comparisons. Such tasks are called logic operations. For example, overtime pay must be credited to those employees who work over forty hours in one week. The task would be to compare the employee's "hours worked" field to 40. If the "hours worked" is greater than forty, the program would multiply time and one-half for all hours worked over forty. There are many situations in a business or agency where comparisons are necessary, if data are to be properly processed.

Procedures

It is extremely important to remember the computer system that is used will be shared by employees, and that written procedures are necessary to facilitate the smooth interface between users. There must be procedures for system users, system operators, and system designers. The system users may not be computer professionals. In this case, a procedures manual must be available which describes HOW to use the system, WHO can use the system, and HOW input data are prepared. Furthermore, unauthorized use must be prevented while the computer system is being developed.

The procedures must cover what happens during normal working situations, but yet users must also know what to do if the computer system is down (not functioning). For example, what happens to the normal daily computer routine if there is a thunderstorm and the flow of electricity is stopped for an extended period of time? Are manual procedures to be used? Should all transactions be stopped while the computer is inoperable? What procedures are to be followed during this difficult time? These issues must be addressed before difficulties arise.

Systems operators (usually computer professionals) must also be informed of proper procedures. They must know when programs are to be run, who has the authority to operate programs, and the form input will assume. Further, there must be written procedures that detail the procedures to be followed when a programmer writes programs for the organization.

It is critical that computer operators know the procedures to follow during crises situations. For example, if the electricity is interrupted while the computer is processing a program, everything in the memory of the CPU may be lost. The computer operator has to plan ahead for this contingency. How can lost data be recovered? One solution is that the computer operator should be required to make back-up copies of all data files and programs. This is one strategy that will make the procedures for unusual circumstances easier to handle.

It should be stressed that the procedures to be followed must be written and available to all employees in the form of a policy manual. Employees should not be allowed to handled the computer until they fully understand operational procedures.

Personnel

Computer personnel can be divided into three types: system designers, operations personnel, and users. System designers include computer programmers and systems analysts. In large organizations, several system designers may be necessary. However, in small agencies these jobs may be handled either by software companies or computer consultants.

Operations personnel include those persons who keep the computer functioning, shut it down for routine maintenance, make proper back-up copies of files, and, in general, understand how the computer physically functions.

The third category of personnel relates to the user(s) of the system. As mentioned earlier, these persons may not have had any formal training with regard to using computers. Nonetheless, many times a person is required to utilize a computer on a job without knowing anything about how this device functions. It is necessary, therefore, that these users receive in-service training to understand the computer system. For example, the person who uses a 24-hour bank teller machine is using the bank's computer system. Therefore all instructions must be easy to read and follow.

Even though the system's users do not know about the computer's internal operation, they still need to know what to do when the system fails. If an agency uses a computer to do initial interviews, what should be done if the system goes down? Waiting until this situation occurs is far too late to decide actions. If an agency is small, one person performs all of the initial interview tasks. If that is the case, computer classes may be the answer to the computer novice's problems.

Security

It is necessary to consider the physical security of a computer system, as well as the safety of the data that are stored. Getting unauthorized information out of a computer system should be made difficult.

There are several types of computer crimes committed: theft of data, theft of programs, damage to a computer system, and the invasion of private data records. It is the responsibility of the computer professional to guard against the invasion of computer data by unauthorized persons.

Maintaining the confidentiality of data is important. Information on practically every person appears in numerous data banks, such as those operated by social security, Internal Revenue Service, educational institutions, banks, credit lending institutions, and more. All citizens are guaranteed the right of privacy by the Fourth Amendment to the Constitution of the United States. The delivery of data concerning a person, without his or her permission is illegal.

If an organization holds information on the people it serves, this information must be kept confidential. There are various ways to secure this data, including physical security mechanisms and the use of passwords.

Basically, using a password means that a person who tries to extract data from the computer banks must first know a code (words or numbers), before the computer will allow access to the data. It is also the responsibility of the organization to keep secure the password. The more confidential the data, the more strict the security needs to be. When computers were first available, people were so pleased with the easy accessibility of data that they forgot information might also be stolen.

In discussing physical security, consideration must be given to the physical placement of the computer in the building. For years, large organizations were so proud to be able to afford a computer that they placed it behind glass walls for everyone to see. As far as security is concerned, that is the worst location for a computer. It should be in the basement, behind locked doors.

Controlled access to the computer room is a necessity. It only takes one disgruntled employee, with a strong magnet, to destroy every secondary storage file. A password or code should be necessary to enter the computer room, but only those who are authorized should have access to this area.

Some thought must also be given to the acquisition of software. Many computer crimes relate to this process. Most of the software that is available for sale is copyrighted and must be purchased from a software dealer. The theft of computer software is a very serious problem. Everyone is tempted to obtain the software at the lowest possible cost. However, the author of a software package may feel quite different. In order to be ethical, a fair price must be paid for computer software.

Developing a New System

The procedure for developing a new system involves a definite cycle of events. Each computer system must fit into the agency requirements of several people. Therefore, developing a system is not easy.There are five major steps to the system development cycle: 1) preliminary investigation, 2) detailed system analysis, 3) system design, 4) system development, and 5) system implementation and evaluation.

Before beginning this cycle of events, a committee must be formed to study the situation. The committee does not necessarily have to be comprised of computer professionals. This group should include persons directly involved with the proposed system, management personnel, and some persons who are knowledgeable about computers.

During the preliminary investigation, the purpose is to find out if there really is a problem that a computer might be able to solve. The proposed problem may originate from a disgruntled employee or management level personnel - someone believes there is a problem. To find out whether the problem is real, or if an employee is just having a bad day, a systems analyst or other management person would go to the department involved and just ask a few questions. A personal interview with the employees involved should reveal whether there is a problem or not.

At the end of each of these steps, a report is provided to management. The report will either state that there is no problem, or there is a problem that warrants a full-scale systems analysis.If management is convinced that a problem does exist, the systems development committee begins to work on Step 2, a detailed systems analysis. During this second step, the committee uses personal interviews and questionnaires to determine how the present system works and how it might be improved.

As journalists like to say, the following questions are asked: who? what? when? where? why? and how? Most importantly, however, WHY a job has been done a certain way must be addressed. Many times the answer comes back: "We've always done it that way!" Once the detailed investigation has been completed, a presentation will be given to management with recommendations for one or more approaches to solving the problem.

One question that must be answered during this phase of system development is whether or not a computer can help solve a problem. Many problems are not computer related. In the absence of computer expertise, a computer consultant may be needed. However, an organization may already have staff persons who will be valuable during this analysis.

So far, no money has been expended other than that of salaries for the committee members and possibly for a consultant. Once management has approved the development of a new system, monetary expenditures are likely to follow. Most important, no analysis should be undertaken without the support of management, not only financial support, but philosophical support as well. A new computer system will cause many changes in the workplace, changes which often cause "people problems." The new system is doomed to fail without strong management support.

Once management has given the green light, Step Three - System Design - can be inaugurated. This task is very time consuming, for it involves the step-by-step development of a new system. Input records, files, the data base, and processing methods must be designed. The format of the output report must also be formulated, so that appropriate reports are produced. Before the report format is formulated, the system's users should be asked to provide input. It is important to note at this juncture that the systems analyst or computer consultant cannot do this job alone. Potential users of the new system must be involved early in its design. No computer consultant has the knowledge or experience to know how each department works. These experts must rely on the department personnel to provide this information.

For example, if the payroll department is to be computerized, the people who work in that department should be asked, "What jobs would you like the computer to be able to do for you?" What reports are time consuming? What about payroll checks - do you want the computer to print payroll checks each week? What data are necessary for the reports you send to the Internal Revenue Department?

During this design stage is when decisions are made about the type of input, type of secondary storage (magnetic tape or magnetic disk), amount of data needed, and the style of output required (computer terminal screen only or printed report), as well as the size and type of computer hardware to be used. While this stage may require months of planning, no aspect should be overlooked.

As in steps 1 and 2, a report is supplied to management at the end of the design stage. Difficult decisions will now have to be made regarding the expenditure of money. Is the organization willing to expend the money to put this new system into action?

If management has given its support for the proposed system, Step 4 involves development. The purchase of hardware and software, along with hiring new personnel and/or training old staff persons, occurs at this time. This, too, is a very time-consuming step. If, for example, ten new microcomputers have been ordered for the payroll department, weeks might pass before they are delivered. Some things just cannot be done quickly. If computer programs are to be written, this is very time consuming as well.

It is important to remember here that drastic changes may be made in the way things "have always been done" in an agency. Many times those changes can be handled very well by the computer, but the problems that result are usually "people problems". If a secretary's typewriter is to be replaced by a computer terminal, this change may cause problems. The people affected should be included early in the planning stages, because they are then more likely to support the new system.

It is also important to point out that management approval is vital during system development and implementation. Invariably, there will be employees who do not like the new system and complain. This is the time when management must support the new system and let an unhappy employee know that this system is here to stay. Suggestions from that employee are always welcome, of course.

Once management approval has been given to proceed further, Step 5 - System Implementation and Evaluation can be undertaken. During this stage, hardware is actually wired into the system, software is purchased and tested, employees are trained, and the system is actually set into operation.

There are several ways to implement a new system. One is to plunge right in, and on a particular date stop the old system and begin the new one. This is very dangerous, because there are always "bugs" which need to be worked out in a new system. It would be wiser to use a parallel system which allows the use of the new computer system while continuing the old system for a period of time. This causes duplication in work effort but is well worth the effort, because a "safety net" is provided in case the new system does not work as planned. If a system has been well planned and designed, there should be few problems.

No one should forget to evaluate the new system. Questions must be answered regarding how well the new system fits the requirements first stipulated in the analysis stage. How close to the budget were the expenditures? What problems still exist? Did the company get the most for its money? All of these questions and more must be reviewed in a final report to management after the system is implemented.

It is not uncommon for the development of a new computer system to take from one to two years. Do not rush this process. Every aspect of the problem must be analyzed so that the outcome will be a system that works to generate the desired output.

The Technological versus the Social System

As should be recognized from the foregoing discussion, many non-technological issues are related to the successful design and implementation of a computer system. In fact, emphasizing technological concerns may not foster the development of management or diagnostic systems. Using computer technology, in other words, requires that many non-technical factors be addressed. The following represent some of these considerations.

1. A program should have clearly defined goals and objectives. In this way, the types of information, number of reports, and the reasons why data are collected can be unambiguously stipulated.

2. The sources of data must be determined. Accordingly, barriers are identified, both in terms of personnel and organizational structure, that may prevent the collection of data.

3. An organizational structure should be established that allows information to be gathered and disseminated. A management style that is authoritarian, for

example, may not facilitate this process. Sharing information must come to be viewed as beneficial to the members of different departments.

4. Planning committees must be established for the purpose of determining how the management reports that are generated will be used. In the business community these groups are referred to as "key report" committees. The idea of this practice is that producing additional data does not necessarily guarantee better management. Data must be profitably used.

5. Training must be provided both before and after a system is chosen. Likewise, managerial and social supports must be provided, so that employees are not intimidated by the new computer system. Computers should also be chosen with their users in mind. For example, a system that is overly complex may never be used effectively, although technically it can do almost an unlimited number of tasks.

6. The context in which computers are to be used must be taken into account. An in-take department is usually a hectic place to work. Therefore, a computer system that is not easy to operate — that is, is user-friendly, quick, and flexible — may never be mastered or useful.

7. Both managers and workers should be prepared to cope with the social changes the introduction of computers will likely spawn. Procedures for voicing complaints and proposing remedies for problems should be formulated. Managerial and organizational strategies to deal with change productively should be instituted.

8. Workers must sense immediately that their jobs will be improved through the adoption of computers. Therefore, every attempt must be made to illustrate both the positive and negative implications of computer use. In this way, rational planning can be undertaken.

At this juncture, the aim is not to be exhaustive, but to indicate that computer systems operate in the midst of social systems. Unless this point is recognized, the use of computers may be dysfunctional to an organization. Therefore, a significant amount of effort should be devoted to integrating the computer and the social system. The promise of high-tech should not blind managers or line staff to the social basis of computerization.

SUGGESTED READING

Austin, Charles J., (1983), *Information Systems for Hospital Administration*, Health Administration Press, Ann Arbor, Michigan

Christensen, William W. and Eugene I. Stearns, (1984), *Micro-computers in Health Care Management*, Aspen Publications, Rockville, Maryland

Clowes, Kenneth W., (1982), *The Impact of Computers on Managers*, UMI Research Press, Ann Arbor, Michigan

Enger, Normal L., (1976), *Management Standards for Developing Information Systems*, AMACOM, New York

Garrett, Raymon D., (1976), *Hospital Computer Systems and Procedures, Vol. I, Accounting Systems*, Petrocelli/Charter, New York

Garrett, Raymon D., (1976), *Hospital Computer Systems and Procedures, Vol. II, Medical Systems*, Petrocelli/Charter, New York

Hodge, Melville H., (1977), *Medical Information Systems*, Aspen Systems Corporation, Germantown, Maryland

Kelly, Joseph F., (1970), *Computers and Management in a Changing Society*, McGraw-Hill, New York

Schmitz, Homer H., (1979), *Hospital Information Systems*, Aspen Systems Corporation, Germantown, Maryland

3

Practical Computer Applications in the Psychotherapy Process

John S. Wodarski, Ph.D.
Associate Vice President of Research and Graduate Studies, The University of Akron

The 1980's can be characterized as the decade of information accumulation and organization, as a result of the incorporation of computer technology into daily activities (Butterfield, 1983; Schoech, 1982; Taylor & Gibbons, 1981; Toffler, 1980). This social and political phenomenon has emphasized the necessity of providing human services on the basis of data. Data provide the rationale for the planning and delivery of services and their subsequent evaluation, along with fiscal support for current and future endeavors. Today, status among human service agencies is determined to some degree by the number of computers and the amount of data that is collected. Unfortunately, however, agencies in many cases are collecting data without an adequate conceptual rationale. Thus the relevance of the technology to human services programming is reduced.

Agencies are finding that resources are no longer the prohibitive factor in the introduction of computer technology. However, as is the case in all fields, application of this technology often lags behind its development. This manuscript addresses the development and implementation of data management systems pertinent to the provision of appropriate services by psychotherapists.

The applications of computer technology relate to a wide range of problems and administrative tasks. One major area of application is that of information management for expediting the delivery of services to clients. Agencies are finding computers to be tremendous timesavers in compiling service statistics, processing payrolls, and preparing financial reports. Moreover, computer technology makes possible forms of inquiry that were heretofore inconceivable, particularly since the computer permits more timely and expeditious use of sophisticated research techniques on routinely available data. Specific applications of computer technology in the performance of managerial, clinical, research and training tasks are presented next.

MANAGERIAL APPLICATIONS

Paper work consumes an inordinate amount of time and energy in traditional human service agencies. The computer's word processing capability dramatically decreases paper work in the production of reports, letters, memos, payrolls, tests, and forms. Once a draft of a document is available, there is a significant reduction in time needed to modify it. Tailoring different reports from the same store of information, outlining plans for worker development, and preparing budgets are other useful applications. In tight financial times, computer applications can facilitate an agency's billing, financial screening procedures, review and revision of fee schedules, and maintenance of accounts to buffer cash flow problems (Goplerud, Walfish, & Bruskowski, 1985). Through word processing all of these functions are completed in record time (Boyd, Hylton, & Price, 1978).

CLINICAL APPLICATIONS

Client Descriptive Analyses

All agencies require data to describe their services. These data provide a rationale for the agency budget and help in the planning for future needs. With appropriate data intake forms, information can be retrieved quickly and accurately to determine: (1) who is served, (2) duration of services, (3) cost of services, (4) who provided the service, and (5) follow-up. Thus, agencies can use this data for soliciting program support and documenting the services that have been rendered. Once such a system is functional, an agency can engage in a variety of analyses of cost effectiveness. This requisite of practice, so evident in the 1980's, provides agencies with a means for making decisions regarding the maintenance or expansion of desired services (Catherwood, 1974; Rapp, 1984).

Numerous concrete items can be easily computerized regardless of the practice context. Contracts executed between client and worker can be checked for the inclusion of the following: purposes of the interaction, targeted problems and areas of difficulty to be worked on, goals and objectives, client and therapist duties, delineation of administrative procedures or constraints, techniques to be used, duration of contracts and criteria for decisions on termination, and renegotiation procedures (Wodarski & Bagarozzi, 1979). Goal-setting forms which specify the type of client difficulty, plans for therapy, short- and long-term goals, plans for termination, and follow-up procedures provide documentation to facilitate the evaluation of progress made toward meeting treatment goals that fulfill legal requisites. A summary form can be used to specify an overall treatment plan, including termination and follow-up procedures (Carlson, 1985; Green, 1985; Meldman, Harris, Pellicore, & Johnson, 1977).

Computers likewise can improve evaluation through checking to see if practice notes summarizing the major events of the client's last visit are recorded within a reasonable time frame, such as 72 hours after each session, and determining if the following are executed when necessary and placed in the client's record expeditiously: letter to referring professional regarding treatment plans and diagnosis, summary of termination notes and follow-up procedures, and, if necessary, a letter to the referring professional or family doctor regarding the termination of services within one week after termination. In all instances the time and energy required for executing the forms should be kept to a minimum (Rinn & Vernon, 1975. Requisite clinical tasks are facilitated by the computer's ability to keep records current and readily available.

Diagnosis, Treatment Planning, and Documentation of Program Implementation and Effectiveness

Many personal computer systems aid in the administration of various assessment inventories and interview schedules. These provide relevant historical data on which clinicians can base their assessments and plans for subsequent treatment (Hedlund, Vieweg, & Cho, 1985). Computer assessment and interview schedules are available for almost all commonly seen disorders (Butcher, 1987; Schwartz, 1984).

National Computer Systems Professional Assessment Services, Institute for Personality and Ability Testing, Inc., and Creative Evaluations are just a few of the organizations capable of scoring assessment inventories in the areas of (1) abnormal personality, (2) normal personality, (3) behavioral health and medicine, and (4) aptitudes and career/vocational interests. For example, the following are available: Adjective Checklist, Bender Visual Motor Gestalt Test, California Psychological Inventory, Career Assessment Inventory, Clinical Analysis Questionnaire, The Exner Report for the Rorschach Comprehensive System, General Aptitude Test Battery, Giannetti On-Line Psychosocial History, Guilford-Zimmerman Temperament Survey, Hogan Personality Inventory, Millon Adolescent Personality Inventory-Clinical, Millon Adolescent Personality Inventory-Guidance, Millon Behavioral Health Inventory, Minnesota Multiphasic Personality Inventory (MMPI) Basic Service, MMPI-The Minnesota Report: Adult Clinical System, MMPI-The Minnesota Report: Personnel Selection System, Multidimensional Personality Questionnaire, Myers-Briggs Type Indicator, The Rorschach Comprehensive System, Self-Description Inventory, Sixteen Personality Factor Questionnaire, Strong-Campbell Interest Inventory, Temperament and Values Inventory, Vocational Information Profile, and Word and Number Assessment Inventory. For an extensive review of the tests that are available consult Ben-Porath and Butcher (1986).

RESEARCH APPLICATIONS

Fuller (1970), in discussing the utility of computer simulations for research, asserts that computer technology is now within the range of almost every practicing psychotherapist. Access to a computer and programs is as near as the extension service of a university's computer center. Even so, the literature regarding direct application of this technology to the agency and practitioner levels remains sparse (Wodarski, 1986).

Computers are essential for research purposes. Once information is organized and placed in the computer, complicated calculations become routine. Transformation of data, simple graphing of client goals, and modification of data for larger analyses are facilitated. The frequently used SPSS is now available in software for personal desktop computers. This innovation increases the practitioner's ability to execute relevant basic statistical analyses of cases. Thus, in general, the ability to analyze the richness of clinical phenomena is enhanced. However, as with all technology, one must have an adequate conceptual rationale as to why certain analyses are relevant.

TEACHING PSYCHOTHERAPY SKILLS BY COMPUTERS

A man-machine model of simulation includes interaction with a machine, usually a computer. Simulation is defined as the process of representing and/or modeling the behaviors of a system on a computer, whereby the software model attempts to mimic the processes of the original system as closely as possible. For example, in the education of psychotherapists, students enter data in the model, the student's input is acted upon, and the system responds with previous programmed responses. In computer simulations, all of the features of a real system are reduced to the highest degree of abstraction, with corresponding logical decision rules and operations which are then programmed for computer manipulation (Meinert, 1972).

The field of computer technology is blossoming at a staggering rate. In fact, the computer is becoming so important that unless a student becomes familiar with them he/she is destined to be unsuccessful in both school and the workplace (Green, 1984). Most important is that computer interaction be required in the education of a psychotherapist.

Computer technology entered the psychotherapy profession in the early sixties, with the exploration of ways to use technology in counseling. By 1970, two annotated bibliographies and two small volumes were written on the use of computer technology by counselors. However, during the 1960s and 1970s the computer was seen as an assistant to the counselor, and programs that taught problem solving skills and provided information were designed. Recently, informational and diagnostic data bases have been developed, along with models of systematic interventions, mechanical clients with which to practice, and supervisory monitoring systems (Phillips, 1984a). As the use of the computer continues to make inroads into the helping professions, the need to include their use in education increases (Alpert, 1986).

The computer has inherent value for education, apart from the need to know how to use it in the work place. Phillips (1983) discusses the attractiveness of computers for education in the tasks and methods of individual instruction. A computer can be seen as an intelligent tutor, thereby reducing the student-teacher ratio. Fascination with the medium is another plus. Increased study time and greater learning may be induced. There are two ways a computer can help a psychotherapy trainee with skills acquisition. First, there is didactic presentation, which includes examples of the skill. Second, there is simulation (Phillips, 1984b). The use of a computer as a simulator has been compared to that of a cadaver for surgeons.

Programs are now being written for the general public, which can be used by or adapted to the education of psychotherapists. These programs are called "life enrichment software" or "psycheware programs", and are designed to accept decision responses from one or more people. The programs allow multiple branching sequences. These programs include *Eliza*, which simulates a nondirective therapist; *Mind Prober*, which estimates another person's attitudes; *Childpace* and *Discover Your Baby*, intended to produce improved parenting; *Coping with Stress* and *The Party*, which teach the adolescent about the effects of alcohol; and *Mr. Howard: A Behavior Therapy Simulation* involving a client referred to a community mental health for anxiety-related complaints (Lambert, 1987). Finally, *Skip* is a highly interactive program that allows the user to learn about aspects of his or her own personality. According to White (1984), there are enormous possibilities for the use of computers in therapist education. There is also a danger, however, to the general public in these "self-help" programs. White compares them to the "self-awareness groups" of the sixties. Hence, psychotherapists must be familiar with these types of programs.

Simulated Psychotherapist

To be of most use to the education of psychotherapists, programs must be interactive. Interactive programs have multiple branching-out contingencies, which are dependent upon the responses of the user. To be effective, the computer must be able to understand the client's natural language. The program must also be able to follow a therapeutic plan when dealing with a client. This can be problematic, but inroads into research on artificial language have been made. *Eliza*, for example, simulates a nondirective therapist. This program analyzes each statement typed into the computer and then responds with a question or comment. This program is limited, however, for it can not recognize nonsense and lacks intuition (Agras, 1987; Weizenbaum, 1966).

Morton is a computer-assisted therapy program that deals with the shortcomings of *Eliza. Morton* deals with a related psychological problem and offers particular treatment strategies. Using a variety of cognitive and behavioral therapeutic techniques, *Morton* deals with depression. It uses multiple choice items and case vignettes to aid the user in the identification of dysfunctional thoughts. Those thoughts are analyzed that are assumed to be the major source of depression (Wagman & Kerber, 1984). Yet another interaction program is *PLATO Dilemma Counseling System* (PLATO DCS). This program is designed for the treatment of avoidance-avoidance problems. Dilemma counseling and the solution of cognate problems is the focus of attention.

As these programs are designed to teach people how to deal with various issues, trainees can learn how to teach people by using a computer. Because these programs must be exact, trainees can learn therapeutic processes precisely. The programs facilitate learning because they are patient, reliable, and efficient. Trainees can also experience what their future clients may feel like by using these systems.

Simulated Clients

The preceding programs all take on the role of the therapist. These simulations are helpful in teaching a student exactly "how to" conduct a therapy session. However, there are other programs that simulate a client and allow the trainee actually to practice his or her skills. One such program, as described by Lichtenberg (1984), is called INTERACT. The assumption behind this program is that counseling is social interaction. Therapy consists of a series of verbal and/or nonverbal exchanges. The INTERACT program analyzes the counselor-client transactions, or response contingencies. It helps trainees learn how to elicit certain classes of responses, which have been shown to contribute to favorable counseling outcomes. Also developed by INTERACT is an awareness of the impact those responses have on clients, in addition to how a therapist's actions may be shaped by a client.

Another fascinating program described by Lichtenberg, Hummel, and Shaffer (1984) is CLIENT 1. CLIENT 1 simulates client behavior during an initial intake interview. The model client is a 30-year-old verbal, motivated, and not overly resistant man. There are several topics that the client can talk about, but they are not all of equal importance. Only one is his primary concern. Each topic is ranked from general to specific, while each statement is ranked according to threat value. The counselor's task is to get the client to verbalize about a specific and threatening aspect of his problem. Progress is defined as moving towards specificity and threat. The strength of the counseling relationship, e.g., the level of trust, is continually reevaluated by the computer. It is determined by the accuracy and appropriateness of the counselor's response. If the trainee continually makes inaccurate or inappropriate judgments, a low "good counselor average" will occur and the session will be prematurely terminated.

This type of program has many uses in the education of psychotherapists. It is flexible and allows variables to be altered, thereby facilitating the recognition of negative counseling habits. Counseling skills can be broken down into their component parts and analyzed. Clients can be made simple or complex, and will not be harmed by the trainee's mistakes. This will allow the trainee to see the value in simply reflecting until good data are available. Finally, a trainee can move back to any portion of the interview and play the game "what if I had said...". This option, which can be invaluable, is not available on any other training medium.

Videodisc Simulation

In making the transition from informal to laboratory modeling simulations, the point should be made that phases of development are being discussed rather than distinct conceptual categories. The transition to what the literature refers to as "laboratory simulation" seems to indicate an increase in structure, or complexity of a task, which the earlier developed informal simulations lacked.

As technology has become more sophisticated, and people have begun to be more creative, many new educational tools have become available. Interactive video is one such tool. Iuppa (1984) defines interactive video as any video system in which the sequence and selection of messages is determined by the user's response to the material presented. The design of video simulation should include as many real images as is possible. He points out that interactive video allows learners to see the consequences of their choices, and thus is the real strength of this type of learning medium.

Growing out of the interactive simulations with the micro computers, videodisc simulations are somewhat more realistic. Prior to the videodisc there were interactive videotape programs. In fact, there are even computer languages and software packages that will allow a person, who knows absolutely nothing about programming languages, to create an interactive simulation (Hosie & Smith, 1984). These include the use of a video cassette recorder, but they are cumbersome and not very practical. Since they do not have random access to any segment of the recorded material, as is the case with discs, video cassettes are very slow. However, with the disc's greater sophistication, there is not much in the way of course work that could not be converted into a computer-controlled interactive videodisc (Pribble, 1985). The big difference between this type of computer-based simulation and instruction is that the videodisc has the ability to simulate reality.

Videodiscs allow a fast and random access to any part of the disc in less than a second. Discs hold up to 54,000 single video frames per side, and can accommodate up to 30 minutes of moving imagery. Of course, the micro computer controls access, evaluates responses (as in the CLIENT 1 program), displays text, and even asks questions. Hence, the trainee can learn verbal and nonverbal skills before working with actual clients.

There is some evidence of the effectiveness of videodisc training (Pribble, 1985). In 1984, the University of West Florida trained a group of welfare department employees in the administration of food stamps, using a 16-hour interactive videodisc course. The trainees finished the training course 25% faster than the control group, which was taught in the traditional manner. Also, 66% of the interactive group passed the posttest, while only 50% of the control group passed this exam.

There is an authoring system for interactive computer simulations that can be adapted to simulations in the education of psychotherapists. The hardware and software of the authoring system was developed by the staff of the Interactive Videodisc for Special Education Technology (IVSET). Five criteria were adopted by IVSET in developing the system for the education of mentally retarded children. First the programmer should be able to use the system regardless of computer experience, while, second, flexibility of instruction should exist. Third, the system should collect data to analyze. Fourth, a teacher should be able to author a program. And, fifth, the system should be capable of summarizing data and monitoring a students progress (Thorkildsen, 1982). This system is fairly easy to use. All that is required is time, energy, and little creativity. Given the benefits of simulation, many programs should be developed. The Interactive Technology Groups, based in Santa Fe, New Mexico, has developed a five-disc course on human relation skills (Pribble, 1985). Hence, a beginning has been made into this exciting and promising field.

In summary, computers can assist psychotherapists in attaining the following goals:

1. Administration and scoring of tests
2. Interpretation and reporting
   a. Wechsler
   b. Rorschach
   c. MMPI
3. Client program planning and evaluation
   a. goals
   b. case progress
   c. intervention plan
   d. timetable
4. Program documentation
   a. data recording and illustration
   b. data analysis
   c. meeting legal and administrative requisites

5. Research applications
   a. client progress
   b. calculations
   c. transformation of data
   d. graphing client and administrative variables
   e. frequency updating of information in data base
6. Teaching psychotherapy skills
   a. client assessment
   b. building relationships
   c. choosing treatment interventions
   d. simulating the psychotherapy process
   e. practicing implementation of criteria for termination
   f. developing maintenance procedures

DEVELOPING A SYSTEM

The development of a computer system requires a knowledge of needs and of what the system may be expected to do. Prior to the selection of any particular computer system the following questions must be addressed: What type of data are needed? What kind of software is available to meet these needs? What forms will be necessary to collect the necessary data for analysis? Who will collect the data? How will the data be stored? How will confidentiality of the data be insured? Will a data specialist be needed? How can one insure that the appropriate individuals are involved in setting up the system and in its subsequent use?

An assessment of financial and time resources is the next step, which is followed by a review of both needs and resources with others knowledgeable about informational systems. If available, a number of different management systems should be studied. Various experts should be enlisted to help. Evaluate what they are doing with their systems and ask others who are working with the system. Visit a similar agency, in which an information management system is already operational. Pilot test the system before full scale implementation. Read journals that now have sections devoted to the latest computer applications to human service delivery (for example, *Computers in Human Behavior*, *Computers in Human Services*, the *Behavior Therapist* by the Association for the Advancement of Behavior Therapy, and *Behavioral Assessment*).

Agencies must avoid becoming infatuated with products pushed by enthusiastic salespersons or in-house "experts." In the words of Crow and Odewahn (1987):

The lack of technical expertise within many human service organizations has led to the creation of specialized units of 'computer experts' who are responsible for the system. These experts frequently 'approach problems differently, use different languages, and have different goals' (Kirtisch & Weisbord, 1977, p.6) from those of the personnel who will be using the output from the system. The orientation of these 'computer people' is usually toward the hardware and unique applications, while the 'users' are generally oriented toward clients and the solution of their individual problems. The resulting communication problem usually leads to frustration for both groups and to the very real possibility that the system will be ineffective (p. 101)

The management information system should be as simple as possible, or "user friendly". Most human service personnel are not going to become computer specialists, so the system should avoid the use of complicated person-computer interactions pertaining to software preparation and time to access the system.

Crow and Odewahn (1987) elucidate four steps to help ensure the success in designing and implementing an effective management information system.

The manager, to avoid as many problems as possible, must (1) understand the workings of the current information system, (2) determine information needs and priorities, (3) ensure maximum organizational input into the development of the system, and (4) ensure that the system is understood by organizational personnel (p. 103).

Informational Requisites

The first requisite in developing an informational management system is to determine how the data will be collected and what assessment instruments and forms are necessary. It is essential that the collected data be reliable and valid.

Second, it is essential that the agency considers the number of files that will be necessary for the collection of such data. The more files needed, the more complicated the management in accessing the files and the more costly. The files also should be evaluated in terms of how much data they will contain, will they interface with other systems, and can the central processing unit handle the numbers.

Individuals who develop the data system must determine how many files should be free-form versus fixed-form format. Free-form records are used to document client assessments, treatment, and follow-up. They are rich in descriptive information; however, they are more difficult to condense and summarize. For example, if a practitioner wishes to view all cases of potential suicide, the computer can be instructed to review all case documents and list cases where this potential is indicated. Such an analysis is slow and costly.

A fixed-form record specifies the exact nature of the data to be collected. A typical example would be a structured interview schedule used to secure descriptive data on clients. The computer can summarize quickly the number of clients for a specific service period in terms of age, income, marital status, and number of children (Kreuger & Ruckdeschel, 1985).

Employee Support and Training

Employee support must be enlisted prior to the institution of an informational management system. The involvement of as many staff as is feasible should take place at the earliest possible date. Easy physical access and instructual modeling will facilitate employee use. Emphasis should be on making joint decisions with regard to the type of records needed. Finally, the agency must determine who will have access to the data and implement appropriate security measures to maintain confidentiality. Securing the file is relatively simple in light of the technological developments in access coding (Naisbitt, 1982).

ISSUES AND IMPLICATIONS

The preparation of psychotherapists with knowledge about computers can be used to help clients is essential (Lawrence, 1986; Sampson, 1986). Clearly, the client change process and the interventions used to help clients are complex. Zastrow (1985) elaborates the intricate interactions:

At this point there is some support (although much research is needed) for the notion that changing negative or irrational self-talk is the key therapeutic agent in psychotherapy approaches. If accurate, the old argument of which therapy approaches are effective and which are not (Eysenck, 1952; Stuart, 1970) may in the near future be refocused to "Which therapy approaches are most effective in changing negative and irrational self-talk?" and "How can present therapy approaches be refined, and new approaches developed, to more effectively change negative and irrational self-talk? (p. 504)

Computers can facilitate the understanding of these processes, and thus enhance the ability of a therapist to tailor appropriate computer assisted interventions to enhance a client's strengths.

To be truly effective, the human service field must come to grips with defining outcomes and standards for service. When outcomes are ambiguous, their standardization is impossible and data comparisons across agencies are meaningless. Informational systems can be utilized to plan and implement agency goals. For example, computers can (1) facilitate an empirically oriented approach to the identification, collection, organization, and analysis of data about clients; (2) aid in the study of the component processes and outcomes of human service delivery systems; (3) clarify the state of the human services in terms of needs; and (4) facilitate the evaluation of different theories of behavioral change and intervention. At the national level, a data system might be developed that would lead to the isolation of how the policies of governments, both federal and state, affect client functioning.

Even if information management systems become readily available and agencies implement them, technical expertise will be necessary to aid in the interpretation and summarization of the knowledge gained from the systems. Moreover, experts should be prepared to summarize the data and disseminate them to other agencies that deal with similar clients. Such a process will add to the knowledge base of the human services.

Sufficient time should be spent initially in setting up an adequate system since it is much more difficult and costly to change a data system once it is operational. Compatibility among systems to increase their utility should be addressed. For example, client diagnosis and treatment plans in mental health agencies might be compared to those of clients in family service agencies. Finally, it is suggested that a yearly evaluation of an informational management system be conducted. The evaluation should include how professionals will use the system, types of information to be collected, and how the organization will be structured to facilitate the use of the data.

Preparation of this manuscript was facilitated through a special projects grant funded through the Office of the Vice President for Research, University of Georgia Research Foundation; the general operating budget of the University of Georgia School of Social Work and the Institute for Behavioral Research; and by awards from the National Institute of Mental Health, Social Work Education Branch MH13753 and MH17208.

REFERENCE NOTE

1. Addresses for these organizations can be secured from the author or by consulting *The APA Monitor* (American Psychological Association newsletter) or *Behavior Therapy*.

REFERENCES

Agras, W. S. (1987). Presidential address: So where do we go from here? *Behavior Therapy, 18*, 203-217.

Alpert, D. (1986). A preliminary investigation of computer-enhanced counselor training. *Computers in Human Behavior, 2*(1), 63-70.

Ben-Porath, Y. S., & Butcher, J. N. (1986). Computers inpersonality assessment: A brief past, an ebullient present, and an expanding future. *Computers in Human Behavior, 2*(3), 167-182.

Boyd, L. H., Jr., Hylton, J. H., & Price, S. V. (1978). Computers in social work practice: A review. *Social Work, 23*(5), 368-371.

Butcher, J. N. (Ed.). (1987). *Computerized psychological assessment*. New York: Basic Books, Inc.

Butterfield, W. H. (1983). Computers: An overview. *Practice Digest, 6*(3), 3-5. Carlson, R. W. (1985). Connecting clinical information processing with computer support. *Computers in Human Services, 1*(1), 51-66.

Catherwood, H. R. (1974). A management information system for social services. *Public Welfare, 32*(3), 56-61.

Crow, R. T., & Odewahn, C. A. (1987). *Management of the human services.* Englewood Cliffs, NJ: Prentice-Hall.

Eysenck, H. J. (1952). The effects of psychotherapy: An evaluation. *Journal of consulting Psychology, 11*, 319-324.

Fuller, T. K. (1970). Computer utility in social work. *Social Casework, 51*, 606-611.

Goplerud, E. N., Walfish, S., & Bruskowski, A. (1985). Weathering the cuts: A delphi survey on surviving cutbacks in community mental health. *Community Mental Health Journal, 21*(1), 14-27.

Green, M. S. (1984). Computer resources and terminology: A brief introduction. *Counselor Education and Supervision, 24*(2), 133-141.

Hedlund, J. L., Vieweg, B. W., & Cho, D. W. (1985). Mental health computing in the 1980's: Part one: General information systems and clinical documentation. *Computers in Human Services, 1*(1), 3-33.

Hosie, T. W., & Smith, C. W. (1984). PILOTING. *Counselor Education and Supervision, 24*(2), 176-185.

Iuppa, N. V. (1984). *A practical guide to interactive video design.* White Plains, NY: Knowledge Industry Publications.

Kirtisch, R. S., & Weisbord, M. R. (1977). Getting computer people and users to understand each other. *Advanced Management Journal*, Spring, 5-14.

Kreuger, L. W., & Ruckdeschel, R. (1985). Microcomputers in social service settings: Research applications. *Social Work, 30*(3), 219-224.

Lambert, M. E. (1987). MR. HOWARD: A behavior therapy simulation. *The Behavior Therapist, 10*(6), 139-143.

Lawrence, G. H. (1986). Using computers for the treatment of psychological problems. *Computers in Human Behavior, 2*(1), 43-62.

Lichtenberg, J. W. (1984, April). *A computer program to assist counseling trainees in understanding interpersonal influence processes in their counseling.* Paper presented at the annual meeting of the American Educational Research Association. (ERIC #248426)

Lichtenberg, J. W., Hummel, T. J., & Shaffer, W. F. (1984). CLIENT 1: A computer simulation for use in counselor education and research. *Counselor Education and Research, 24*(2), 155-167.

Meinert, R. G. (1972). Simulation technology: A potential tool for social work education. *Journal of Education for Social Work, 8*(3), 50-59.

Meldman, M. J., Harris, D., Pellicore, R. J., & Johnson, E. L. (1977). A computer-assisted, goal-oriented psychiatric progress note system. *American Journal of Psychiatry, 134*(1), 38-41.

Naisbitt, J. (1982). *Megatrends.* New York: Warner Books.

Phillips, S. D. (1983). Trends and implications for training: Counselor training via computer. *Counselor Education and Supervision, 23*(1), 20-28.

Phillips, S. D. (1984a). Computers as counseling and training tools. *Counselor Education and Supervision, 24*(2), 130-132.

Phillips, S. D. (1984b). Contributions and limitations in the use of computers in counselor training. *Counselor Education and Supervision, 24*(2), 186-192.

Pribble, R. (1985). Enter the videodisc. *Training, 22*(3), 91-99.

Rapp, C. A. (1984). Information, performance and the human service manager of the 1980's: Beyond "housekeeping." *Administration in Social Work, 8*(4), 69-80.

Rinn, R. C., & Vernon, J. C. (1975). Process evaluation of outpatient treatment in a community mental health center. *Journal of Behavior Therapy and Experimental Psychiatry, 6*(1), 5-11.

Sampson, J. P., Jr. (1986). An integrated approach to computer applications in counseling psychology. *The Counseling Psychologist, 11*, 65-74.

Schoech, D. (1982). *Computer use in human services: A guide to information management.* New York: Human Sciences Press.

Schwartz, M. D. (Ed.). (1984). *Using computers in clinical practice: Psychotherapy and mental health applications.* New York: Haworth Press.

Stuart, R. B. (1970). *Trick or treatment.* Champaign, IL; Research Press.

Taylor, J. B., & Gibbons, J. (1981). *Using microcomputers in social agencies.* Beverly Hills: SAGE Publications.

Thorkildsen, R. (1982, March). *Microcomputer/videodisc authoring system for instructional programming.* Paper presented at the annual meeting of the American Educational Research Association. (ERIC #227841)

Toffler, A. (1980). *The third wave.* New York: Bantam Books, Inc.

Wagman, M., & Kerber, K. W. (1984). Computer-assisted counseling: Problems and prospects. *Counselor Education and Supervision, 24*(2), 142-154.

Weizenbaum, J. (1966). ELIZA—A computer program for the study of natural language communication between man and machine. *Communications of the Association of Computing Machinery,9,* 36-45.

White, A. (1984, October). *A sample of counselor educators about microcomputers.* Paper presented at the annual meeting of the Northern Rocky Mountain Educational Research Association. (ERIC #253811)

Wodarski, J. S. (1986). The application of computer technology to enhance the effectiveness of family therapy. *Family Therapy, 13*(1), 5-13.

Wodarski, J. S., & Bagarozzi, D. A. (1979). *Behavioral social work: An introduction.* New Your: Human Sciences Press.

Zastrow, C. (1985). *The practice of social work* (2nd ed.). Homewood, IL: Dorsey Press.

4

Computer-Assisted Psychological Assessment and Intervention

Sharon W. Foster
Department of Pediatrics and Staff Psychologist, University of Wisconsin, Hospital and Clinics

Harold P. Erdman
Lead Systems Analyst, Health Care 2000, Laguna Honda Blvd., San Franciso, CA

Concern over the rising costs of health care has led to increased attention to ways to provide more cost-effective treatment. Psychological factors have been implicated as contributing to a substantial proportion of health care costs. A number of researchers have suggested that between 50 and 75 per cent of primary care *medical* visits may involve psychosocial factors (Hellman, 1984). These figures must be considered, in addition to the number of persons who come directly to mental health care providers for assistance. Crucial to curtailing health care costs is that psychosocial issues be identified and receive appropriate treatment. Among the more innovative responses to these concerns has been the development of computer programs to aid in assessment and intervention with persons with psychiatric/psychological dysfunction. Although such programs cannot replace the mental health professional, they offer considerable potential for improving the delivery of mental health services in a cost effective manner.

As has been discussed previously, computer-assisted psychological assessment and intervention offers a number of potential advantages (Erdman & Foster, 1986; Erdman, Klein, & Greist, 1985; Greist & Klein, 1980; Greist, Klein, Erdman, & Jefferson, 1983,). Among these advantages are: 1) potential for wide availability, 2) a balance of consistency and flexibility, 3) patient acceptance, and 4) competitive cost-effectiveness.

First, computer-assisted intervention programs can be readily disseminated. Microcomputers have been increasingly employed in mental health settings. Their use, however, has been confined primarily to administrative tasks, such as billing and record management. Clinical applications have related predominantly in scoring personality or other assessment inventories. The potential exists for assessment and intervention programs, reflecting current expertise, to become available to the increasing number of clinicians having microcomputer technology. More importantly, clients would be able to benefit from expertise not locally accessible. The potential is thus for a wider range of clients, in diverse settings, to benefit from assessment and intervention approaches not previously available.

Second, such programs offer a balance of consistency and flexibility. These programs reliably perform the designated interventions with patients for whom a mode of treatment has been judged appropriate, regardless of other patient characteristics (such as age, or socio-economic status), time of day, location, or other factors not immediately germane to treatment outcome. They will also consistently carry out each component of the treatment as designated, e.g., conducting an assessment of any change in the client's symptom status, following up on homework assignments, providing psychoeducational information, and other requisite tasks. This standardization also affords researchers the opportunity to evaluate treatment that is standardized to a degree rare in human intervention, and thus allows outcome evaluation and treatment modification based on empirical evidence. Computer-assisted assessment and intervention also permits flexibility in responses to the client, although acknowledgeably to a lesser extent than human therapists. A number of programs reviewed in the following section permit branching, depending on the nature of a client's responses. Currently, programs branch from such relatively circumscribed subprograms as the representation of an item on desensitization hierarchy (Biglan, Villwock, & Wick, 1979), to exploring the client's expectations about treatment when s/he has indicated non-completion of a homework assignment (Selmi et al., 1982). The potential flexibility of computer-assisted treatment is vast.

Third, computer-assisted psychological assessment and intervention shows promise of high client acceptance. Previous research on client attitudes towards computer-assisted assessment has suggested high patient acceptance, with some studies even suggesting that some patients prefer computerized assessment over that conducted by a human interviewer (e.g., Evan & Miller, 1969; Slack & Slack, 1977; Slack & VanCura, 1968). Research has also suggested that subjects may reveal more information to a computer than to a human interviewer, particularly on what clients may view as emotionally laden topics such as sexual functioning, drug/alcohol use, or suicidality (Carr, Ghosh, & Ancill, 1983; Griest & Klein, 1980; Lucas, Mullin, Luna, & McInroy, 1977). A related benefit may occur as a function of the extent to which the programs allow clients to see themselves as active agents in their own change process. This may be true particularly of persons who, because of socioeconomic status or cultural background, may tend to feel judged or intimidated by a mental health professional whose characteristics on such factors may be dissimilar (Johnson & Mihal, 1973).

One other issue bears note. A number of commentators have suggested that computer psychotherapy is inherently fraudulent, in that the essential ingredient of any psychotherapy is the experience of an interpersonal connection with another human being. That view is not contested here: A number of caveats on use of computer-assisted psychotherapeutic intervention are discussed in the last section of this chapter. At the same time, we believe it is unethical to withhold treatment, the efficacy of which has been established, from those who would benefit from it. As will be reviewed in this chapter, there have been a wealth of studies that evaluate the effectiveness and patient-acceptance of computer-assisted assessment and intervention programs. These studies have shown overwhelming positive outcomes. Several trends, including national concern about the rising costs of health care, the increased percentage of care provided in the context of prepaid health care organizations (HMO's, IPA's, EAP's, etc.) and the concern about cost containment associated with such groups, concern about potential cutbacks in federal funding for health care programs, and increased attention within the mental health field itself to the development of shorter-term, focused psychotherapeutic intervention (e.g., Strupp, 1981) augur well for the increased development of more cost-effective treatments. Computer-assisted assessment and intervention programs may provide one way of addressing this need. While concern about such programs is great, this concern may likely spur researchers to meet the challenges by developing programs which meet high levels of demonstrated effectiveness.

The aim here is to sketch the history of these efforts, describe current developments, and offer a critique of the methodological and ethical issues involved in the use of computers in providing mental health care. In addition, recommendations will be offered for future developments.

COMPUTER-ASSISTED ASSESSMENT

Computer-administered data gathering, of which computer-based psychological testing and assessment is one example, began with the work of Slack, Hicks, Reed & Van Cura (1966). Their work offered a computer-based medical history interview. The interview exhibited sophisticated branching capabilities, as well as direct prompts to patients to aid their progress through the interview. Evaluation of the reactions of over 300 patients to the system was highly encouraging. This pioneering contribution paved the way for subsequent developments in computer-assisted assessment.

In two decades since the initial work by Slack and his colleagues, interest in, and development of computer-assisted assessment has burgeoned. Such programs have been based on widely-used paper-and-pencil instruments such as the Minnesota multiphasic personality inventory (MMPI), as well as on interview protocols. The primary advantage of the computer in this area is its ability to combine the strengths of standard paper-and-pencil instruments with some of the intelligence and flexibility of a human. Since a program performs exactly as instructed, a computer guarantees total reliability in its questioning process, never forgetting a question and always following the same format. As a result, computerized assessment has the potential for being more complete than other modes of evaluation. Indeed, Carr, Ghosh, & Ancill (1983) found that a computerized psychiatric history obtained, on the average, 5 1/2 items per patient that were not recorded by the treating clinician, including such clinically significant facts as having a criminal record (26%) or attempting suicide (17%). Standardized questionnaires provide the same benefit, but the computer can also provide flexibility by differentially responding to the client's input. While still far removed from the capability of the average person, the less a skilled clinician, the computer's ability to follow up with additional questions when a client indicates a problem in one area, or to insert earlier responses into the client's record when doing a more detailed examination, make it a more interactive and exciting medium than written questionnaires.

There are other advantages to using a computer that are especially relevant to testing and assessment. Computer administration enhances data integrity. A computer can prevent incomplete questionnaires by repeating or rephrasing a question until a response is given. A computer can be programmed to accept only valid responses for a particular question, thus preventing incorrect input. Validity checks can be performed, and key questions may be repeated if inconsistent responses are obtained. Finally, by obtaining results in a directly computer-compatible form, computerized test administration facilitates computer scoring, especially of long and complicated instruments. No transcription or recording of responses is necessary, thus eliminating one potential source of errors.

Two dimensions along which computer-based assessment can be categorized are: 1) the content area of the assessment instrument, and 2) the degree to which the program is interactive. While the value of instruments that can incorporate flexible branching have been emphasized, such systems require more development.

Indeed, the simplest way to create a computer-based instrument is to computerize an already existing standard questionnaire. A critical research question in this case is to ensure that the computer instrument has the same psychometric properties as the paper-and-pencil questionnaire on which it is based. A common example of such a computer-administered test is the MMPI (e.g., Lushene, O'Neil, & Dunn, 1974; Johnson & Williams, 1974; Johnson & Williams, 1980; White, Clements, & Fowler, 1985). Typically, high correlations and comparable mean scale scores are found between computer and standard paper-and-pencil administration. This trait of comparability has been found with other standard instruments, including the Beck Depression Inventory, and Trait Anxiety Inventory (Lukin, Dowd, Plake, & Kraft 1985), the Marital Adjustment Test (Parks, Mead, & Johnson, 1985), and the

Wechsler Adult Intelligence Scale (Elwood & Griffin, 1972).

However, as indicated earlier, the computer-based instruments with the most promise are those that go beyond standard questionnaires, and use the computer's flexibility in branching. In some cases, this may involve developing new instruments specifically for the computer. An example of such an instrument developed specifically for computer administration is a suicide risk prediction interview (Greist et al., 1973; Erdman et al., 1987). An example of the branching capabilities relates to asking detailed questions about a previous suicide attempt if one has been made, but skipping over these items if the client has never before attempted suicide. In a retrospective evaluation, where both clinicians and the computer made predictions based on written case histories, the computer was more accurate that the clinicians (Greist et al., 1973). While clinicians' performance improved when they evaluated patients actually under their care, the computer was at least as accurate as the clinicians (in fact, somewhat more accurate, but the overall difference was not statistically significant) (Erdman et al. 1987).

An assessment concept that depends on the computer's branching ability is adaptive testing (Vale, 1981; Weiss, 1985). By varying the number and specific items used, i.e., by selecting as the next test item the one that is most appropriate to the trait level of the individual, it is possible to obtain more precise trait estimates, while still using fewer items than with a fixed set of items on a questionnaire.

An assessment program based on an already existing instrument, but utilizing the computer's branching ability, is the computer version (Greist et al. in press) of the diagnostic Interview Schedule (DIS) (Robins, Helzer, Croughan, & Ratcliff, 1981). In this case, of course, the reason why the computer program utilizes sophisticated branching is not because it is replacing paper-and-pencil instrument, but rather one-administered by a human. By allowing use of the DIS without utilizing skilled clinician time, training, or interviewing staff, the computer extends the capability of practicing clinicians to obtain highly standardized, completely structured, and relatively comprehensive diagnostic data. Additional research on the computer program revealed that its reliability is comparable to that of the human-administered DIS. Some examples of other systems using branching include programs for psychiatric history-taking (Maultsby & Slack, 1971), alcohol consumption assessment (Lucas, Mullin, Luna, & McInroy, 1977), and phobia assessment (Carr & Ghosh, 1983).

COMPUTER-ASSISTED INTERVENTION

In addition to being used to assist in psychological assessment, computer programs have also been developed to assist in actual psychotherapeutic intervention. The following overview illustrations the diversity of such applications, as well as summaries of studies on the effectiveness of computer-assisted interventions. While further research clearly needs to be conducted, the data to date suggest that these programs show promise as adjuncts to more conventional psychotherapy approaches.

Early developments

One of the seminal, albeit unintentional, triggers to the development of computer-assisted psychological intervention was Weizenbaum's (1966) program ELIZA. Crudely modeled on some principles of Rogerian psychotherapy, ELIZA exhibited the ability of the computer to identify key words or phrases, and make certain transformations on the input. ELIZA was created with the purpose of demonstrating the technical capabilities of the computer to respond in a limited way to a restricted set of features of natural language communication. ELIZA has been cited, however, as an example of computers perceived by human users as capable of understanding and responding to human thought and emotion. Weizenbaum (1976) subsequently forcefully argued against this interpretation of ELIZA's or any other computers capabilities.

In the same year, Colby and his associates (Colby, Watt, & Gilbert, 1966) announced the development of a program that was explicitly aimed at providing interaction that the user would experience as psychotherapeutic. The program functioned by identifying keys (characters, words, or phrases) in the subjects' input, responding via teletype by either producing a response matched to the key word or phrase, or by putting the key word or phrase in a context designed to elicit further input (e.g., asking the subject "why do you feel x"?). The program also kept track of input for later use, including new keys. Another function of the program was to respond differentially depending on whether a key appeared in the subjects input in the beginning, middle, or end of a "session". Colby et al. reported that at the time of their report, the program was perceived as frustrating to users. They suggested that future development would need to include a significantly larger dictionary of both input keys and responses, as well as greater program flexibility. They also offered the intriguing recommendation that researchers consider not only modeling programs on current psychotherapeutic practice, but also investigate models of unique contributions to be offered by computer client-interaction.

Lang (1969) was among the first to apply computer technology to the modification of a specific behavioral dysfunction, that of phobias. He described a Device for Automated Desensitization (DAD), a system that involved several functions; 1) instruction and muscle relaxation, 2) a previously collected hierarchy of fear-arousing stimuli, and 3) a series of behavioral interventions, including instructions on imagining fear-arousing material, relaxation, and inquiry about the degree of the subjects fear response. Physiological data were collected concurrent with the subjects' interaction with DAD. The subject controlled the progression through the hierarchy by a switch located on his/her chair. Subsequent modifications allowed a more detailed inquiry of the subject's visualization, as well as instruction techniques to increase visualization, as well as instruction techniques to increase visualization skills. Other changes included concurrent analysis of physiological data, and expanded stimulus presentation capabilities. Lang's later research, discussed in the following section, offers strong evidence for the potential for computer-assisted intervention in the treatment of specific behavioral dysfunctions.

These and other early demonstration projects, using what by present-day standards would be considered cumbersome technology, demonstrated the therapeutic benefit to be derived from human-computer interaction. First, they provided evidence that individuals were willing to describe personal problems to a computer, even though at that stage subjects reported frustration with the interaction. In fact, research by Slack and Vancura (1968) suggested that some patients might present more personal information to a computer than to a human interviewer. Second, these demonstration projects suggested that if a problem area could be described with sufficient detail, a computer could collect data useful for future subject-computer interaction. Colby's et al. incorporation of new keys and Lang's use of physiological monitoring are both examples of this capability. Third, these researchers illustrated that the computer could exhibit flexibility in responding to subjects, depending on the subject's input. This was a crucial demonstration, which showed the potential for computer-assisted interaction to address a particular individual's needs, in addition to allowing interaction to be controlled by the subject.

Recent Developments

In the two decades following the early demonstration projects there has been an explosion of interest and effort in the development of computer-assisted psychological intervention. For comparison purposes, these have been grouped here by area of application.

Anxiety Disorders. One of the major applications has been to the treatment of anxiety disorders, particularly various phobias. These computer aids have been readily applied in this area, due to the relatively greater specificity of treatment methods for such disorders and greater consensus among clinicians about the appropriate components of treatment programs.

Lang and his colleagues (Lang, 1980; Lang, Melamed, & Hart 1970) have presented strong evidence for the utility of a systematic desensitization procedure for phobias. Using an updated version of the program described above, Lang, et al. (1970) conducted an outcome study comparing three groups; 1) a DAD treatment group, 2) one in which desensitization was administered by a human therapist, and

3) a no-treatment control group. Results suggested that subjects treated with DAD exhibited comparable and, on some measures, superior outcomes to subjects treated by a human therapist. DAD-treated subjects also maintained improvement as well or better than human therapist treated subjects,eight months following treatment. These impressive results argue favorably for the utility of the DAD automated desensitization procedure.

A group at the Institute of Psychiatry in London have published a series of reports on computer-assisted assessment and treatment of phobias (Carr & Ghosh, 1983a; Carr & Ghosh, 1983b; Ghosh, Marks, & Carr, 1984; Ghosh & Marks, 1987). Their automated treatment program, modeled on the work of Marks (1978), is aimed at aiding the subject in graduated *in vivo* exposure to a fear stimulus, and utilizes homework assignments and involvement with the subject's significant other in the treatment process. The program, as described by Ghosh, et al. (1984), consists of four major components: 1) a phobia assessment, 2) treatment planning, 3) weekly assessment and review, and 4) outcome and follow up. Earlier research (Carr & Ghosh, 1983a, 1983b,) suggested that the assessment component of the program was highly correlated with a human evaluator. This was particularly true regarding the identification of persons with agoraphobia and social phobia, although inadequate number of cases of other phobias were available to permit statistical comparison. The treatment components of the program were evaluated in an outcome study comparing psychiatrist, automated, and self-help treatment groups (Ghosh & Marks, 1987).

Subjects were all diagnosed as agoraphobic, with reported mean duration of dysfunction of nine years. Results indicated that all three treatment groups exhibited statistically significant improvement from pretreatment to posttreatment, and that all groups showed maintenance of improvement at a 6 month follow-up examination.

Several reports have described the use of computer-assisted treatment programs for persons with test anxiety. Biglan, Villwock, & Wick (1979) reported the development of a program consisting of audio taped relaxation training and computer-assisted desensitization techniques. Subjects were trained in relaxation prior to beginning the desensitization procedure. The desensitization component was comprised of a standard hierarchy of 20 items pertaining to test anxiety.

The automated test anxiety program was evaluated by an uncontrolled outcome study. Methods of evaluation included the Suinn Test Anxiety Behavior Scale, clinical interviews, and subjects' ratings of discomfort during test-taking situations. Results provided evidence for the utility of the computer-assisted program in reducing testing anxiety, with subjects exhibiting changes from pre-treatment to post-treatment in test anxiety. The authors did not, however, specify the statistical significance of their findings.

A program for computer-assisted assertiveness training was reported by

Muehlenhardt (1981), based on previous work by McFall and his colleagues (McFall & Lillesand, 1971; McFall & Marston, 1970; McFall & Twentyman, 1973). The program incorporates widely accepted principles of assertion training, including coaching, modeling, rehearsal, and corrective feedback. Muehlenhardt's program consists of two components. The fully automated program was compared with two other treatment groups semi-automated audiotaped training and fully automated audiotaped training and a motivation-only control group. Results suggested that all three treatment groups showed improvement on various measures of assertiveness and their improvement was significantly different than controls.

Affective Disorders. Self-reported depression is one of the most common complaints of persons seeking mental health treatment. It is therefore noteworthy that two programs have been developed for computer-assisted treatment of depression. These programs are appropriate only for persons who have been evaluated and diagnosed previously as exhibiting mild to moderate depression. Selmi (Selmi, Klein, Greist, Johnson, Harris, 1982) developed the most comprehensive treatment program for depression to date. The program, dubbed MORTON, was based on the cognitive-behavioral intervention principles proposed by Beck (Beck, 1976; Beck, Rush, Shaw, & Emery 1979). MORTON consists of 6 to 8 sessions, each 40-50 minutes duration, designed to be administered over a 6 week period. The first session consists of attempts to establish rapport, addressing expectations of therapy, eliciting major complaints, providing information about cognitive-behavioral principles and assigning homework. With each session, the Beck Depression Inventory (BDI) (Beck, Ward, Mendelson, Mock, & Erbaugh, 1961) is also administered. The second session includes introducing agenda setting, reviewing, and clarifying previously covered material. Session three includes computer-assisted agenda setting, a didactic presentation of material on dysfunctional automatic thoughts, and instructions which enable the subject to identify his/her own dysfunctional cognitive distortions. The following sessions proceed through more advanced stages of identifying cognitive distortions, while providing education on how to develop more rational thought processes and guidelines for managing future depressive episodes.

MORTON was evaluated in a study comparing a human therapist, MORTON, and treatment on demand (control) groups (Selmi, Grist, Klein, Sorrell, & Erdman, unpublished manuscript). The group led by a human therapist was conducted using a protocol essentially similar to that adopted by MORTON. Thirty six subjects, who met research criteria on a number of instruments widely used to measure depression, were randomly assigned to one of three groups. Subjects were assessed pre-treatment, post-treatment, and at two months following up treatment on the SCL-90 (Derogatis, Lipman, Rickels, Uhlenhuth, & Covi, 1974), The Hamilton Rating Scale-Depression (HRS-D) (Hamilton, 1960), Automatic Thoughts Questionnaire (ATQ) (Hollan & Kendall, 1980), and BDI. BDI scores from each of the six session administrations were also used. Results suggested that there were no statistically significant differences between the computer-assisted and human therapist groups. Also suggested was that both treatment groups improved more than control group subjects.

Lawrence (1981, 1986) described a more circumscribed, but potentially valuable, program aimed at increasing the utility of homework assignments, as an adjunct to cognitive-behavioral therapy for depression. The program describes a cognitive-behavioral view of depression and associated treatment, items designed to assess the subject's comprehension of the material, and assessment of and feedback on the client's assertiveness, using a scale based on the work of Lazarus (1971). The program also presents logs for mood and behavior. These are included to promote self-monitoring and provide insight to the client about his/her cognitive-behavioral patterns.

Problem-solving and Educational/Vocational Counseling. Wagman (Wagman, 1979, 1980; Wagman & Kerber, 1980) has developed an innovative program for aiding clients in clarifying and resolving difficulties in making choices. The dilemma counseling techniques on which the program is based were designed to be applicable to a wide range of client difficulties, including problems of a personal nature as well as more conventional educational/vocational ones. The program, after an introduction into the system, guides clients through 5 steps; 1) formulating the problem as a conflict between 2 choices, and specifying the aversive consequences for each, 2) determining an "out" for each of the choices, 3) rephrasing the question in a more creative way that permits possible positive outcomes, 4) generating solutions for each of the above creative inquiries, and 5) ranking and evaluating the solutions. The program, PLATO-DCS, was designed to be used on the PLATO system, originally developed at the University of Illinois at Urbana/Champaign, with terminals available nationwide and in Canada.

Evaluation of PLATO-DCS included users' assessments of their personal acceptance of computerized counseling, and their evaluation of PLATO-DCS as 1) a teacher of methods of problem-solving, and 2) a personal counselor in helping them with their own difficulties. Seventy-seven subjects were randomly assigned to either the PLATO-DCS group or to a no-treatment control group. Methods of assessment included a 22-item questionnaire asking subjects to rate their perceptions of their personal acceptance of this system, the teaching effectiveness of this system, and the counseling effectiveness of the system. Results suggested that subjects viewed PLATO-DCS as helpful both in terms of teaching problem solving skills and helping them with personal difficulties. Subjects also indicated preference for PLATO-DCS, as compared with a human counselor, further, the majority disagreed with the statement that the system was "too impersonal". Also, upon follow-up, the PLATO-DCS group showed "a greater reduction in problem troublesomeness as compared with a control group" (Wagman, 1980, p. 26). Further evaluation of PLATO-DCS essentially supported these findings (Wagman, 1982; Wagman & Kerber, 1980).

Sampson (1983, 1986; Sampson & Stripling, 1979) has discussed the use of computers in counseling interventions, and specific applications to educational/vocational choice. He has distinguished between information systems and guidance systems. Information systems aid clients in identifying characteristics of a desired career, and obtaining information about careers that meet the desired characteristics. Guidance systems provide a broader range of functions, including help in clarifying job-related values, developing plans for the future, and evaluating the likely success of those plans.

Intervention programs have also been developed to provide assistance in more specific areas such as study skills (Sampson, 1981), health risk appraisal (Raines & Ellis, 1982), and value clarification (Rokeach, 1975). Other areas that have been suggested as areas for further development of counseling intervention programs include: assertiveness training, conflict resolution, communication skills, social skills, parent training, and stress management (Sampson, 1983).

Weight management. A computer-assisted therapy for obesity was developed and tested by Burnett, Taylor, and Agras (1985, also see Agras, 1987). The treatment program provides on-line behavioral treatment of obesity via a portable microcomputer. The computer program requires clients to self-monitor food consumption at meals and snacks, and exercise duration and exertion level. The program calculates total calories for each meal or snack based on input data, as well as total caloric intake that day and the remaining calorie allotment for the day.

Evaluation of the treatment program was conducted by comparing subjects treated by the computer-assisted program and those treated by a similar program using paper-and-pencil methods of self-monitoring. Results showed that the computer-assisted treatment group showed larger weight change during the 8 weeks of treatment (larger magnitude of effect). Follow-up checks at 24 weeks and 40 weeks suggested that the computer-assisted group maintained and even continued weight loss, whereas the control group exhibited some relapse during that same time period. The investigators noted that the results for the computer-assisted treatment group compared favorably with treatment methods using more complex weight loss regimens.

Sexual Dysfunction. Binik, Servan-Schreiber, Freiwald, and Hall (unpublished manuscript) have developed a program for a difficulty that at first glance might seem an unlikely application of computer assisted treatment, that of sexual dysfunction. Their program, Sexpert, demonstrated the feasibility of developing an "intelligent dialogue based examination and treatment expert system". Sexpert first introduces use and limitations of Sexpert, then gathers basic background information on the couple (or individual), conducts an assessment of the clients' difficulties, provides a diagnosis and discusses factors which may be contributing to the sexual dysfunction, and offers treatment for one dysfunction. An informal evaluation of the program suggested that couples appeared affectively engaged in the interaction with Sexpert, and with each other during the interview. They also reported that at least one couple, during a follow-up discussion at home, expressed concerns following interaction with Sexpert. The authors plan a more formal evaluation of Sexpert's diagnostic accuracy and treatment effectiveness.

Child/Adolescent Behavior Dysfunction. Behavior therapists have been exemplary in developing the specific types of assessment protocols and behavioral foci that lend themselves to computer-assisted assessment in intervention. An excellent review of work in this area has been presented by Kratochwill, Doll, & Dickson (1985). Among the applications discussed was the Behavior Manager (Tomlinson, Acher, & Mathier (1984), an assessment and intervention program for use by classroom teachers. The program utilizes information provided by the teacher about the problematic child behavior, the teacher's preferences for consequating behavior, and the classroom routine to offer a plan of action for teacher intervention. No empirical evaluation has yet been conducted on this program.

A therapeutic computer game to help adolescents learn impulse control has been offered by Clark and Schoech (1983). Designed to incorporate both the principles of play therapy and cognitive behavioral training, the fantasy-adventure type game presents a number of scenarios that provide an opportunity for clients to exert decision-making abilities. Clients could earn points or lose points based on the adequacy of their problem-solving skills at each of the choice points. The program coaches clients in problem-solving skills and in the development of positive self-statements to provide an alternative to impulsive behavior. No formal empirical evaluation of the program has yet been conducted. The authors described anecdotal reactions of clients, parents, and other agency staff that suggested such therapeutic games may be a useful adjunct to more traditional forms of psychotherapy for this age group.

Summary

To date, researchers have demonstrated that computer-assisted assessment and psychotherapeutic intervention programs can be developed that are 1) accepted (and sometimes preferred) by clients, 2) effective in producing therapeutic change, and 3) cost-effective. Hence the question is not the global one of whether such programs can be effective in contributing to therapeutic change, but the more trenchant one pertaining to what types of clients, with which types of disorders, using what therapeutic approaches, and under what conditions will behavioral change most likely occur.

Investigators have generally agreed that such programs are most readily applicable for clients with relatively circumscribed disorders, such as simple phobias, mild to moderate depression, or problem-solving deficits. Communication skills, conflict resolution methods, and stress management are among other areas that have been suggested as possible areas of application. The use of a portable microcomputer is a potentially powerful development that may allow advances in treating not only obesity, but also persons with other disorders in which compliance with treatment is often an issue, such as hypertension and diabetes. Such technology may also prove useful in the treatment currently requires client literacy, and most are written in English. There is, however, no *a priori* reason prohibiting the development of programs with varied language options, or which permit interaction via symbols.

Currently, programs are based on theoretical orientations that are primarily cognitive-behavioral. Cognitive-behavioral frameworks have been particularly useful, for they have yielded assessments and treatment protocols that are well-structured, specific, and permit clearer evaluation of progress and therapeutic outcome than many other theoretical frameworks. Cognitive-behavioral approaches have also been demonstrated to be effective for a wide variety of disorders. The use of play therapy in the development of therapeutic games appears to be a promising approach which merits further attention, particularly for programs designed for adolescents. As discussed previously, the research of workers such as Slack and Slack, (1977) using more traditional psychotherapy approaches, suggest that some patients may find interacting with a more traditionally-oriented program helpful. Pending further developments in AI at least, however, the complexity required of programs responding to more open-ended client input are likely to be prohibitive.

A number of programs have been purported to be fully automated. As will be discussed in the following section, we do not believe that computer assessment or intervention programs should be used on a stand-alone basis. This is due to both the technical limitations of such programs to date and ethical and legal considerations.

The empirical testing and evaluation of computer-assisted assessment and treatment programs is commendable. It should be continued. While well-designed research has been conducted on many of the programs reviewed here, all programs should be considered experimental and subjected to further study. This is especially true given that, for better or worse, computer-assisted assessment and intervention programs are likely to be met with skepticism and close scrutiny for some time to come.

GUIDELINES FOR THE USE OF COMPUTER ASSISTED ASSESSMENT AND INTERVENTION

"Instruction Manual"

This section describes the steps clinicians should use in selecting mental health computer applications. The first step is to have a clear idea of the client's problem, in order to determine that it is one for which a computer-based assessment or intervention is appropriate. In other words, clinicians should not be so enamored of computers that they become like the person given a hammer, to whom every problem begins to look like a nail. While enthusiasm about the potential uses of the computer is warranted, programs do not yet exist that are suitable for most of the problems exhibited by most clients.

In particular, the state of the art is such that treatment programs are currently relevant only to relatively well-defined problems. A worthwhile generic program for psychotherapy does not yet exist and will never exist unless major strides are made in several areas of artificial intelligence, most especially natural language processing. Even the most technologically sophisticated treatment program yet developed (Binik et al. unpublished manuscript) is directed at a relatively specific area of sexual dysfunction. MORTON (Selmi, et al. 1982) is applicable to a relatively large audience, yet the clinician must recognize that the program has only been tested with, and is probably only useful for, those with mild to moderate depression. Those with more severe depression are not good candidates for the program.

The need for a well-defined problem is somewhat less with assessment instruments, as both special purpose instruments, e.g., for suicide assessment (Greist, et al., 1973; Erdman, et al., 1987) and general purpose instruments, e.g. the DIS for psychiatric diagnosis (Greist, et al., in press) exist. However, here too, the clinician still must understand why an instrument is useful and not expect it to do more than it is designed to do. An instrument yielding DSM-III diagnoses may be helpful in suggesting potential treatments for some patients, e.g. anxiety disorders or affective disorders, but it is unlikely to provide direction for a couple seeking marital therapy, except in so far as it screens for the presence of other factors potentially confounded with the marital problems.

Ethical standards require that the clinician uses tested and validated programs, except when the clinician is specifically engaged in research. Both assessment instruments and intervention procedures are being distributed and sold that have not been subjected to any evaluation other than the developer's determination of face validity. Clients should not be exposed to such potentially damaging programs (or indeed, to any unvalidated interventions whether computer-based or not) unless the client is aware of their experimental nature.

The clinician also needs to be sensitive to the client's reactions to the computer system. This does *not* mean discontinuing a program's use at the client's first report of any difficulty or apprehension in using the system. Just as it may be appropriate to encourage client's to remain on tricyclic anti-depressants for at least 3 weeks even though some annoying side effects occur before then, so it may be appropriate to encourage clients to continue with a well chosen computer-based assessment or treatment program despite initial difficulties or misgivings. As indicated earlier, the overwhelming majority of clients *will* respond positively and accept the use of the computer. However, for that small minority who *resolutely* reject a computer program, clinicians should accept the client's decision.

Finally, the clinician must monitor the client's progress with the program, especially for multiple session programs. A client's evaluation of progress should be reviewed to ensure that he or she is proceeding smoothly through the program. If a client's symptomatic status significantly worsens or the client is not complying with the program, human intervention is necessary. The clinician should, thus, only use programs that prepare reports for the clinician documenting these events. If the program is designed to be used by the client alone, without on-going clinical involvement, then the clinician should direct the client to contact the clinician if the program is not proceeding as planned. A well-designed program (and the clinician restricting herself or himself only to tested and validated programs will ensure a minimal level of quality) will have built-in checks that identify situations when the program is not proceeding well and that refer the client to a human clinician.

Ethical and Legal Issues

Ethical and legal issues in the use of computer-assisted psychological assessment and intervention have been addressed by a number of authors (Spero, 1978; Matarazzo, 1980, Zarr, 1984). Although these issues have been reviewed already in some detail (Erdman & Foster, in press), the following summarizes some key concerns:

First, it is imperative that researchers and clinicians not accept *prima facie* claims for the accuracy, comprehensiveness, or effectiveness of computer-assisted assessment or intervention programs. Such programs represent a technological innovation, and as such may be presented with an aura of mystique that may tend to inflate the claims made for them. The American Psychological Association, recognizing potential dangers in the injudicious use of these programs, has published guidelines that address the need for more careful development and employment of such instruments.

Further attention to the development of standards for the development and use of these programs is likely to be forthcoming, as more practitioners explore their utility. In particular, more attention is needed to evaluating the decision rules underlying assignment of diagnoses, test interpretations, and treatment alternatives. To date these algorithms have often been the province of the developer. Further dialogue is essential to achieve a balance between the wish of developers to retain claims to that knowledge (especially when such programs are disseminated on a for-profit basis), and the needs for the discipline as a whole to have such information be in the public domain for purposes of empirical evaluation.

Second, because an assessment or intervention is computerized does not *ipso facto* mean that it is preferable to more conventional methods if administering assessment or treatment. Such programs are only as good as the assessment or intervention methods or principles upon which they are based. Technological advances should not be constructed as substantive advances in theory or technique. Evaluations of such work, therefore, need to be conducted by professionals with a solid grounding in test construction, outcome research, and theories of and approaches to psychological assessment and intervention.

Third, it is unclear, as yet, how third-party payers will respond to computer-assisted work. It is also not clear what legal responsibility is held by clinicians for any potentially deleterious consequences of computer-assisted assessment or treatment. Clinicians clearly do bear *ethical* responsibility for all phases of assessment and treatment, however.

Finally, we recognize that there are many aspects of psychological services that are not yet well understood, and are often relegated to that nebulous realm of "art" rather than science. There are numerous features of human interaction that are simply not "codable" by current computer technology, considering the uniqueness of the individual, his/her history, and present situation. Throughout this chapter the position has been maintained that these programs should be construed as computer-assisted: They are not a substitute for interaction with a human therapist.

REFERENCES

Agras, W. (1987). Eating disorders: Management of obesity, bulimia, and anorexia nervosa. New York: Pergamon.

Angle, H. V., Johnsen, T., Grebenkemper, N. S., & Ellinwood, E. H., (1979). Computer interview support for clinicians. *Professional Psychology, 10*, 49-57.

Beck, A. T. (1976). *Cognitive therapy and the emotional disorders.* New York: International Universities Press.

Beck, A. T., Rush, A. J., Shaw, B. F., & Emergy, G. (1979). *Cognitive therapy of depression.* New York: Guilford.

Beck, A. T., Ward, C. H., Mendelson, M., Mock, J. E., & Erbaugh, J. K. (1961). An inventory for measuring depression. *Archives of General Psychiatry, 4*, 561-571.

Biglan, A., Villwock, C., & Wick, S. (1979). The feasibility of a computer controlled program for the treatment of test anxiety. *Journal of Behavior Therapy & Experimental Psychiatry, 10* 47-49.

Binik, Y. M., Servan-Schreiber, D., Freiwald, S., & Hall, K. S. K. (Unpublished manuscript). Intelligent computer-based assessment and psychotherapy.

Burnett, R. F., Taylor, C. B., & Agras, W. S. (1985). Ambulatory computer-assisted therapy for obesity: A new frontier for behavior therapy. *Journal of Consulting and Clinical Psychology, 53,* 698-703.

Carr, A. C., Ancill, R. J., Ghosh, A., & Margo, A. (1981). Direct assessment of depression by microcomputer. *Acta Psychiatrica Scandinavia, 64,* 415-422.

Carr, A. C., & Ghosh, A. (1983a). Accuracy of behavioral assessment by computer. *British Journal of Psychiatry, 142* 66-70.

Carr, A. L., & Ghosh, A. (1983b) Response of phobic patients to direct computer assessment. *British Journal of Psychiatry, 142,* 60-65.

Carr, A. C., Ghosh A., Ancill, R. J., (1983) Can a computer take a psychiatric history? *Psychological Medicine, 13,* 151-158.

Clark, B., & Schoech, D. (1983). A computer assisted therapeutic game for adolescents: Initial development and comments. *Computers in Psychiatry/Psychology, 5,* 7-20.

Colby, K. M. (1979). Computers simulation and artificial intelligence in psychiatry. In E. A. Serafinides (Ed.), *Methods of Biobehavioral Research,* pp. (145-156). New York: Grune & Stratton.

Colby, K. M., Watt, J. B., & Gilbert, J. B. (1966). A computer method of psychotherapy: Preliminary communication. *Journal of Nervous and Mental Disease, 142,* 148-152.

Derogatis, L. R., Lipman, R. S., Rickels, K., Uhlenhugh, E. N., & Covi, L. (1974). The Hopkins symptom checklist (HSCL). *Behavioral Science, 19,* 1-15.

Elwood D. L. and Griffin R. H. (1972). Individual intelligence testing without the examines: Reliability of an automated method. *Journal of Consulting and Clinical Psychology, 38,* 9-14.

Ekstrom, R. & Johnson, C. (Eds.). (1984). Special Issue: Computers in counseling and development. *Journal of Counseling and Development, 63,* 131-195.

Erdman, H. P., & Foster, S. W. (1986). Computer-assisted assessment with couples and families. *Family Therapy,* XIII, 23-40.

Erdman, H. P., & Foster, S. W. (In press). Ethical issues in computer-assisted assessment. *Computers and Human Services.*

Erdman, H. P., Greist, J. H., Gustafson D. H., Taves J. E., Klein, M. H., (1987) Suicide risk prediction by computer interview: a prospective study. *Journal of Clinical Psychiatry, 48,* 464-467.

Erdman, H. P., Klein, M. H. & Greist, J. H. (1985). Direct patient - computer interviewing. *Journal of Consulting and Clinical Psychology, 53,* 760-773.

Evan, W. M., & Miller, J. R. (1969). Differential effects on response bias of computer vs. conventional administration of a social science questionnaire: An exploratory methodological experiment. *Behavioral Science, 14,* 216-227.

Ghosh, A. & Marks, I. M., (1987). Self-treatment of agoraphobia by exposure. *Behavior Therapy, 18,* 3-16.

Ghosh, A., Marks, I. M., & Carr, A. C., (1984). Controlled study of self-exposure treatment for phobias: Preliminary communication. *Journal of the Royal Society of Medicine, 77,* 483-487.

Greist, J. H., Gustafson, D. H., Stauss F. F., Rowse G. L., Laughren, T. P., Chiles, J. A. (1973) A computer interview for suicide risk prediction. *American Journal of Psychiatry, 130,* 1327-1332.

Greist, J. H., & Klein, M. H. (1980). Computer programs for patients, clinicians, and researchers in psychiatry. In J. B. Sidowski, J. H. Johnson, & T. A. Williams (Eds.) *Technology in mental health care delivery systems* (pp. 161-182). Norwood, NJ: Albex.

Greist J. H., Klein M. T., Erdman, H. P., Bires, J. K., Bass, S. M.,Machtinger, P. E., Kresge, D. G. (In press) Psychiatric diagnosis by direct patient computer interview. *Hospital and Community Psychiatry.*

Greist, J. H., Klein, M. H., Erdman, H. P., & Jefferson, J. W. (1983). Clinical computer applications in mental health. *Journal of Medical Systems, 7,* 175-185.

Gustafson, D. H., Griest, J. H., Strauss, F. F., Erdman, H., & Laughren, T. (1977). A probabilistic system for identifying suicide attempters. *Computers in Biomedical Research, 10,* 1-7.

Hollon, S. D., & Kendall, P. C., (1980). Cognitive self-statements in depression: Development of an automatic thoughts questionnaire. *Cognitive Therapy and Research, 4,* 383-395.

Johnson, D. F., & Midahl, W. L. (1973). Performance of blacks and whites in computerized versus manual testing environments. *American Psychologist, 28,* 694-699.

Johnson, J. H. & Williams T. A. (1980). Using on-line computer technology to improve service response and decision-making effectiveness in a mental health admitting system. In JB Sidowski, J. H. Johnson and T. A. Williams (Eds.). *Technology in mental health care delivery systems* (pp. 237-252). Norwood, NJ: Ablex.

Kratochwill, T. R., Doll, E. J., & Dickson, W. P. (1985). Microcomputers in behavioral assessment: Recent advances and remaining issues. *Computers in Human Behavior, 1,* 277-291.

Lang, P. J. (1969). The on-line computer in behavior therapy research. *American Psychologist, 24,* 236-239.

Lang, P. J. (1980). Behavioral treatment and biobehavioral assessment: Computer applications (pp. 129-138).

Lang, P. J., Melamed, B. G., & Hart, J. (1970). A psychophysiological analysis of fear modification using an automated desensitization procedure. *Journal of Abnormal Psychology, 76,* 220-234.

Lawrence, G. H. (1981). The use of home computers to enhance homework adjuncts to psychotherapy. *Dissertation Abstracts International 42,* 378.

Lawrence, G. H. (1981). Using computers for the treatment of psychological problems. *Computers in Human Behavior, 2,* 43-62.

Lucas, R. W., Mullin, P. J., Lund, C. B. X., & McInroy, D. C. (1977) Psychiatrists and a computer as interrogators of patients with alcohol-related illnesses: A comparison. *British Journal of Psychiatry, 131,* 160-167.

Lukin M. E., Dowd T, Plake B. S., Kraft R. G. (1985). Comparing computerized versus traditional psychological assessment. *Computers in Human Behavior 1,* 49-58.

Lushene, R. E., O'Neil H. F., Dunn T. (1974). Equivalent validity of a completely computerized MMPI. *Journal of Personality Assessment, 38,* 353-361.

Marks, I. M. (1978). *Living with fear.* New York: McGraw-Hill.

Maultsby, M. D., & Slack, W. V. (1971). A computer-based psychiatry history program. *Archives of General Psychiatry, 25,* 570-572.

McFall, R. M., & Lillesand, D. B. (1971). Behavior rehearsal with modeling and coaching in assertion training. *Journal of Abnormal Psychology, 76,* 295-303.

McFall, R. M., & Twentyman, C. T. (1973). Four experiments on the relative contributions of rehearsal, modeling, and coaching to assertion training. *Journal of Abnormal Psychology, 81,* 199-218.

Muehlenhard, G. L. (1981). Comparison of fully and semiautomated assertion training. Unpublished Ph.D. Dissertation, University of Wisconsin, Madison.

Parks, B. T., Mead B. E., Johnson, B. L. (1985) Validation of a computer administered marital adjustment test. *Journal of Marital and Family Therapy 11,* 207-210.

Raines, J. R., & Ellis, L. B. (1982). A conversational microcomputer-based health risk appraisal. *Computer Programs in Biomedicine, 14,* 175-184.

Robins, L. N., Helzer, J. E., Croughan, J. L., Ratcliff, K. S., (1981). National Institute of Mental Health Diagnostic Interen Schedule: It's history, characteristics and validity. *Archives of General Psychiatry 38,* 381-389.

Rokeach, M. (1975). Long-term value change initiated by computer feedback. *Journal of Personality and Social Psychology, 32,* 467-476.

Sampson, J. P. (1983). An integrated approach to computer applications in counseling psychology. *Counseling Psychologist, 11,* 65-74.

Sampson, J. P. (1986). The use of computer-assisted instruction in support of psychotherapeutic

processes. *Computers in Human Behavior 2*, 1-19.
Sampson, J. P., & Stripling, R. O. (1979). Strategies for counselor intervention with a computer-assisted career guidance system. *The Vocational Guidance Quarterly, 27*, 230-238.
Sampson, J. P. (1981). CASSI: A computer-assisted approach to improving study skills. *NASPA Journal, 18*, 42-47.
Selmi, P. M., Griest, J. H., Klein, M. H., Sorrell, S. P., & Erdman, H. P. Unpublished manuscript. Computer-assisted cognitive-behavior therapy in the treatment of depression.
Selmi, P. M., Klein, M. H., Greist, J. H., Johnson, J. H., & Harris, W. G. (1982). An investigation of computer-assisted cognitive-behavior therapy in the treatment of depression. *Behavior Research Methods and Instrumentation, 14*, 181-185.
Sidowski, J. B., Johnson, J. H., & Williams, T. A. (Eds.). *Technology in mental health care delivery systems* (pp. 237-252). Norwood, NJ: Ablex.
Slack, W., & Slack, C. (1977). Talking to a computer about emotional problems: A comparative study. *Psychotherapy: Theory, Research, and Practice, 14*, 156-163.
Slack, W. V., Hicks, G. P., Reed, C. Z., Van Cura L. J. (1966). A computer-based medical history system. *New England Journal of Medicine, 274*, 194-198.
Slack, W. V., & Slack, C. W. (1977). Talking to a computer about emotional problems: A comparative study. *Psychotherapy: Theory, Research, and Practice, 14*, 156-164.
Slack, W. V., & VanCura, L. J. (1968). Patient reaction to computer-based medical interviewing. *Computers and Biomedical Research. 1*. 527-531.
Spero, M. H. (1978). Thoughts on computerized psychotherapy. *Psychiatry, 41*, 279-288.
Strupp, H. H. (1981). Toward the refinement of time-limited dynamic psychotherapy. In S. H. Budman (Ed.), *Forms of Brief Psychotherapy* (pp. 219-242) New York: Guilford.
Tomlinson, J. R., Acher, N. E., & Mathieu, P. J. (1984). *The Behavior Manager*. Minneapolis, MN: ATM.
Vale, C. D. (1981) Design and implementation of a microcomputer-based adaptive testing system. Behavior Research Methods and Instrumentation, 13, 399-406.
Wagman, M. (1979). Systemic dilemma counseling: Theory, method, research. *Psychological reports, 44*, 55-72.
Wagman, M. (1980). PLATO-DCS: An interactive computer system for personal counseling: Further development and evaluation. *Journal of Counseling Psychology, 27*, 31-39.
Weiss, D. J. (1985) Adaptive testing by computer. *Journal of Consulting and Clinical Psychology 53*, 774-789.
Weizenbaum, J. (1966). ELIZA - A computer program for the study of national language communication between man and machine. *Communications of the Association for Computer Machinery, 9*, 36-45.
Weizenbaum, J. (1976). *Computer Power and Human Reason: From Judgment to Calculation.* San Francisco: Freeman Press.
White, D. M., Clements, C. B., Fowler, R. D. (1985) Validation of a computer administered marital adjustment test. *Journal of Marital and Family Therapy, 11*, 207-210.
Zarr, M. L. (1984). Computer mediated psychotherapy: Toward patient-selected guidelines. *American Journal of Psychotherapy, xxxviii*, (1) 47-62.

5

Computer Technology in Clinical Practice:

An Overview of Ethical Concerns

John T. Pardeck, PhD, ACSW
Professor of Social Work, Chair of the Department of Social Work, Southeast Missouri State University, Cape Girardeau, MO 63701

The potential uses of computers in social work practice have expanded dramatically over the last decade. This trend is largely due to recent developments in the field of microcomputer technology. Presently, a complete microcomputer system, including monitor, keyboard, microprocessor, and external storage devices, is readily available at a reasonable price to social work practitioners (Schinka and Smith, 1984).

Even though practitioners appear to be moving slowly toward the adoption of computer technology for direct practice, this trend will probably increase as newer graduates from social work programs enter the workplace (Curriculum Policy for Master's Degree and Baccalaureate Degree Programs in Social Work, 1984). The fields of psychology and psychiatry have been using computer technology extensively for quite some time. Accordingly, a number of studies conducted in these two fields have illustrated that microcomputer technology can be used successfully in several areas of practice, particularly for inventory testing, clinical assessment, biofeedback, word processing, recording, and, in a limited sense, for therapeutic intervention (Pardeck and Murphy, 1986).

The use of computers in clinical practice has not gone unchallenged. A major concern about the use of this technology in the delivery of clinical services is the dehumanization of clients. Specifically, a number of critics have argued that computers remove the human element from service delivery (Hall, 1983). Nevertheless, many of the criticisms that have been lodged against the use of computers have been primarily logistical in nature. In other words, most of the discussions addressing the use of computers in practice have not focused on the ethical issues related to this new technology, especially in the field of social work. Since social workers have been slow to address these important issues, many questions remain

c

to be answered about the impact of computers on the delivery of social services.

The most trenchant critique of the use of computers in clinical practice has been offered by Joseph Weizenbaum (1976), a computer theoretician. Moreover, the social work literature has given little attention to Weizenbaum's criticism of computer technology. The goal of this paper is to expand upon his analysis and address issues that clinical social workers need to begin exploring before the strengths and limits of microcomputer technology can be thoroughly understood. First, microcomputer technology is heavily grounded in quantitative measurement, which means that qualitative approaches to intervention are deemphasized. Second, computerized assessment creates a number of unique problems related to the therapeutic relationship. And third, when computers are used as a therapeutic tool, what happens to the therapeutic discourse?

QUANTITATIVE MEASUREMENT

The language of computers is mathematics. In order for data to be processed, knowledge must be reduced to "bits" of information. This is accomplished through the adoption of binary logic. Binary classification allows information to be inserted neatly into an identification scheme, so that data can be processed and interpreted. As a result of this logic, the data collection process essential to computer processing is standardization. It can be argued, however, that many of the activities done in clinical social work practice are not easily transformed into the logic used by a computer to process information (Gripton, 1983).

A similar position is taken by those social workers who reject the idea that one's practice can be quantified. Central to their argument is that the helping process is so abstract that many practice activities cannot be quantified (Imre, 1984). An example of this would be the difficulty of translating into quantifiable terms the feeling a practitioner has when he or she has established a "positive relationship" with a client. Obviously, some concrete indicators can be identified, such as a client arriving for appointments on time or becoming very verbal during treatment sessions. However, the way a worker defines "a positive relationship" is difficult to measure with respect to precise quantitative indicators.

Another example of the criticisms directed at quantitative approaches to clinical practice would be those lodged against the clinical instruments developed recently by Walter Hudson. Over the past several years, Hudson, (1982) produced nine indexes that measure a number of problems ranging from depression to sexual satisfaction. Hudson's Generalized Contentment Scale, for example, is designed to measure depression. His findings suggest that this scale is extremely valid and reliable. However, those who are critical of quantifiable approaches to practice argue that the twenty five statements, which are structured according to a Likert type scale ranging from (1) "rarely or none of the time" to (5) "most or all of the time", do not appropriately capture the complexities of depression (Hudson, 1982). Recently, Hudson (1985) has extended the development of his indexes to a computer format that allows the client to take the scale sitting at a microcomputer, which in turn scores and interprets a client's responses. Hence instant feedback is provided to the client.

Hudson's work clearly shows the fit between quantitative approaches and the computerization of clinical practice. However, James Gripton (1983) illustrates the link between quantitative approaches and computers by taking the position that before microcomputers can be used in clinical practice, the discursive, non-quantitative interventions which now dominate clinical social work practice will have to give way to therapies based on a strong scientific orientation, such as behavior modification, cognitive restructuring, or task-centered treatment.

The non-quantitative nature of current clinical social work practice suggests that computer technology may present an ethical dilemma for the practitioner. If ethics is viewed as a function of the relationship enacted between the parties involved in a transaction, the introduction of computer technology into clinical practice may result in a practitioner treating a client irresponsibly. The rationale for this conclusion is simple: The qualitative aspect of practice is deemphasized or eliminated (Levy, 1982). In other words, the client may begin to be approached as a source of input, and nothing more. When viewed in this manner, clients are inadvertently objectified.

Even though the fields of psychology and psychiatry have used computer technology successfully for some time in clinical practice, a number of practitioners in these fields have expressed similar ethical concerns about computerized practice. Those with a humanistic orientation toward practice express reservations about computerizing the helping process (Matarazzo, 1983). Although Weizenbaum is not a psychologist or psychiatrist, his arguments most clearly represent the criticisms emanating from these humanists. In his book, *Computer Power and Human Reason*, Weizenbaum (1976) declares that computerized psychotherapy is immoral and obscene, and the sort of activity that "ought to give rise to feelings of disgust in every civilized person." This is so, Weizenbaum explains, because a computer fails to provide interpersonal respect and understanding, not because this device is technically incapable of functioning as an effective psychotherapist.

The point emphasized by humanists is that persons provide themselves and their environment with meaning they produce, through language use and other activities. Unless the logic and reason that is adopted everyday to organize reality can be computerized, the clinical use of computers will not be exceedingly fruitful. In fact, this inability to computerize the cognitive and linguistic assumptions that differentiate fact from fantasy has been a major stumbling block in research on artificial intelligence. Yet if a client's interpretation of reality is ignored, a diagnosis will likely be made in a haphazard manner. Therefore, the humanist's concerns appear to be warranted, at least until the ability of computers to handle natural language has been improved.

This criticism does not mean merely computers must be programmed in language that is recognizable to users. Much more important, the element of interpretation that organizes a client's world must be built into a computer's data base. In other words, the frame of reference presupposed by computerization must be similar to that adopted by those who are studied. As a result, the therapist and client will be able to understand each other's world. Without sensitive interpersonal dialogue, how can therapy occur? This question should not be taken lightly. After all, is the manipulation of overt behavior the same as producing long-term, substantive behavioral change? Behaviorists, for example, may agree with this assessment of therapy, while other, more humanistic practitioners disagree completely with this description of intervention. The aim of therapy, in other words, has a lot to do with whether or not service delivery should be computerized.

COMPUTERIZED ASSESSMENT

The ethical implications of computerized assessment have been explored in a number of articles outside of the field of social work. Most discussions of computerized assessment have focused on computerized clinical testing, interviewing, and the problems related to confidentiality (Hall, 1983, Matarazzo, 1983; Reid and Gorsuch, 1984; Beaumont, 1982).

Few computerized clinical tests have been developed within the field of social work. However, a number of tests are now available in fields of psychiatry and psychology. One key ethical issue concerning computerized assessments is that unqualified persons may utilize test results in an inappropriate way. It has been noted, for example, that computerized tests give the "aura of objectivity" to the untrained user (Reid and Gorsuch, 1984). As a trained clinician realizes, clinical tests must be used with caution and should comprise only one aspect of the evaluation process. Unfortunately, computerized testing systems are being purchased by police departments, employment offices, and other agencies that are not likely to have personnel trained to administer clinical tests. The potential for misuse and, therefore, harm to clients taking such tests is great under these conditions. (Matarazzo, 1983; Hall, 1983).

Even professional practitioners may begin to equate assessment with testing, as noted by Matarazzo (1986). Due to the emphasis placed on science, objectivity, and reliability by technological clinical applications, the *art* of intervention may begin to atrophy. Clinicians must remember that a diagnosis consists of judgments, rather than simply deductive arguments. Computers are deductive, instead of insightful. Yet unless the judgments made by a clinician are socially appropriate, accuracy and consistency may lead to erroneous conclusions. While computers are undaunted by everyday concerns, this sort of uninvolved decision making may be clinically disastrous.

Computerized interviewing is another new development available to the clinical practitioner. The use of the microcomputer for on-line interviewing (primarily to obtain initial intake information or a social history) has not been extensive in social work. However, as the potential for greater use of this technology increases, practitioners must be aware of critical ethical issues related to computerized interviewing.

Erdman et al. (1981) suggests that computerized interviewing is so radically different from traditional forms of interviewing, the role played by the clinician in the interview process must be closely examined. Another major concern with computerized interviewing is that a vast amount of information can be gathered. The result is a mass of confusing facts, which are likely to overwhelm most clinicians. Decision making is thus not enhanced. While this issue may be viewed as mainly a methodological problem, when a clinician's judgments are impaired ethical concerns must be addressed.

Spitzer (1983) argues that the validity of computerized interviewing may be difficult to assess, since this new technology cannot be compared to the usual unstructured interview. A number of articles have reported the problems inherent to placing clients in front of a computer terminal for any reason (Carr, 1982; Skinner and Allen, 1983; Murphy and Pardeck, 1986). As suggested earlier, ignored by a computer program are the factors that supply the context for behavior. Most clinicians would agree that these are key ingredients for successful assessment and treatment. Certainly, a comprehensive assessment must include an examination of a client's milieu. Yet computers do not fare well in this sort of unstructured analysis.

Confidentiality obviously is a major ethical issue when using a computer during the assessment process. There have been a number of recent examples where computer "hackers" have been able to gain access to sensitive information in banks and educational institutions (Burnham, 1980). In terms of clinical practice,if data stored on clients is not properly protected and confidentiality is breached, an important ethical standard is violated. How to insure that information on clients stored within a computer system remains confidential is an important ethical consideration.

In general, through computerization, data come to be viewed as public information. This change has important repercussions for clinical practice. First, the meaning of data is viewed inadvertently to be obvious. Second, the collection of increased information is thought to be beneficial. And third, the secrecy and intimacy usually associated with clinical records seems to dissipate. In other words, clinicians may become desensitized, because every problem is simply an example of a "clinical type" or another variable. Clinicians, nonetheless, should not be lulled into treating their clients dispassionately. The emphasis that is placed on clarity and accuracy must not undermine the passion that is essential for successful advocacy. Someone who is uncommitted may not be a proper advocate.

The question remains: is the acquisition of more data necessarily related to the improved delivery of social services? From a purely technical standpoint the answer is yes.

On the other hand, one piece of relevant information may be more beneficial than a plethora of so-called objective facts. What this suggests is that "communicative competence" is more important than technical skill when making a diagnosis. Increased technical rigor, moreover, does not necessarily lead to communicative or interactive competence. Interaction is a social phenomena that cannot necessarily be created through simulations or other technical means. A clinician must learn to appreciate the pragmatic thrust of a client's language use, before informed discourse is possible. Yet pragmatic questions are anathema to technical ones. The presence of more facts must not blind practitioners to the need for raising pertinent questions.

MICROCOMPUTERS IN *THERAPY*

At MIT during the 1960s, Joseph Weizenbaum and Kenneth Colby developed a program called ELIZA. The ELIZA program is based on a nondirective, Rogerian approach to therapy. It should be noted that ELIZA is experimental and is now largely considered to be a toy. However, research on programs such as ELIZA continues at MIT's Artificial Intelligence Laboratory and elsewhere throughout the world (Weizenbaum, 1976).

The often quoted dialogue that is used to illustrate a typical conversation between ELIZA and a client is as follows:

Client: Men are all alike.

ELIZA: IN WHAT WAY?

Client: They are always bugging us about something or other.

ELIZA: CAN YOU THINK OF AN EXAMPLE?

Client: Well, my boyfriend made me come here.

ELIZA: YOUR BOYFRIEND MADE YOU COME HERE, THAT IS INTERESTING.

Client: He says I am depressed much of the time.

ELIZA: I AM SORRY TO HEAR YOU ARE DEPRESSED.

Client: It is true, I am unhappy.

(Later in the session)

Client: You are afraid of me.

ELIZA: DOES IT PLEASE YOU TO BELIEVE I AM AFRAID OF YOU?

Client: My father is afraid of everybody.

ELIZA: REALLY, EVERYBODY?

Client: My father is very fearful.

ELIZA: WHAT ELSE COMES TO MIND WHEN YOU THINK OF YOUR FATHER?

Client: Bullies.

ELIZA: DOES THIS HAVE ANYTHING TO DO WITH THE FACT THAT YOUR BOY-FRIEND MADE YOU COME HERE?

At first, ELIZA and the client appear to be engaged in dialogue. However, the linguistic limitations of ELIZA become apparent in the following exchange:

Client: Yes.

ELIZA: I SEE.

Client: Yes.

ELIZA: I UNDERSTAND.

Client: Yes.

ELIZA: YOU SEEM QUITE POSITIVE.

Client: Yes.

ELIZA: YOU ARE SURE?

Client: Yes.

ELIZA: I SEE.

Client: Good.

ELIZA: I AM SURE I UNDERSTAND YOU FULLY.

Client: Well, I can't explain.

ELIZA: HOW DO YOU KNOW YOU CANNOT EXPLAIN?

Client:	How does one know anything?
ELIZA:	WHY DO YOU ASK?
Client:	Because I do not know.
ELIZA:	IS THAT THE REAL REASON?
Client:	You are the analyst, you tell me.
ELIZA:	WHAT MAKES YOU THINK I AM THE ANALYST, YOU TELL YOU?

Initially, therapy seemed to be underway in the above dialogue. This is due to the program's ability to make several simple linguistic transformations. The user of the program types in a sentence and ELIZA scans it for the presence of any preprogrammed words. For example, when ELIZA discovers the key word 'alike' in a sentence, this program is designed to respond with the phrase 'in what way?' When the key word 'always' is identified, ELIZA asks for a particular example. When the user answers with the word 'yes,' ELIZA reacts with several canned options. When faced with a neutral statement, ELIZA requests additional information (e.g., "tell me more about it"). Also, ELIZA is programmed to transform certain words reflexively, so that 'you' becomes 'I', 'your' becomes 'my', and so forth.

As illustrated toward the end of the dialogue, ELIZA sometimes makes transformational errors because English is an extremely complicated language. At this time, ELIZA cannot be programmed to account for all the intricacies of language, and thus the dialogue between a user and ELIZA is often non-sensical (Weizenbaum, 1976).

Recent research suggests that computer games may be used effectively as an adjunct to therapy. It has been demonstrated that computer games can help clients to maneuver their way through an imaginary world, comprised of strange creatures and challenging situations. As a player in the game, a client can fight, run, buy, sell, explore, and so on. The decisions made by a client during a game have both long and short term consequences. Ultimately, the decision making process exhibited in a game is translated into real life situations by the therapist.

Certain studies have demonstrated the limited use of computers as a tool in therapy (Reitman, 1984; Barnett, 1984). However, as microcomputer technology advances, and as the potential increases for the use of microcomputers in therapy, two important ethical questions need to be explored: 1) What is it about treatment with a human therapist that is so important? and 2) What differentiates the treatment provided by a computer from that offered by an actual therapist?

The answer appears to lie in the therapeutic relationship itself—that is, the encounter between two human beings in an authentic, genuine atmosphere designed to produce change at the deepest levels of human experience. Sigmund Freud was one of the first therapists to realize that the human encounter is the primary tool for behavioral change. Freud discussed this encounter in terms of the transference phenomena, and this continues to be the core of psychoanalytic treatment (Gill, 1982). Anna Freud appeared to confirm this assumption, as she carried on her father's work. Anna Freud (1954) writes:

> "With due respect for the necessary strictest handling and interpretation of the transference, I feel that we should leave room somewhere for the realization that the analyst and patient are also two real people of equal adult status, in a real personal relationship with each other."

Lewis Wolberg, (1977, pp.31-34), in his classic work *The Technique of Psychotherapy*, outlines the importance of this personal encounter:

> "This (the therapeutic) relationship ideally is a unique interpersonal experience in which the patient feels a quality of warmth, trust, acceptance, and understanding such as he has never before encountered with any human being. Until a working relationship is constituted, the patient particularly will be unable to handle the anxieties associated with unconscious conflict, to resolve repression and other archaic defenses against anxiety, to challenge the spurious protective and pleasure values of his neurosis, and to evolve more constructive modes of personal adjustment...The therapist must provide the patient with an experience that will act as a prototype of a different kind of human relationship—one that inspires new and constructive patterns toward people."

What Wolberg is describing is an atmosphere of change that is only possible between two human beings. That is, the client and the therapist encounter each other authentically, on a variety of levels, and ultimately experience growth and change.

Stanley Strong and Charles Claiborn (1982) emphasize that the therapeutic setting is a social system. Accordingly, interaction and movement within this system produces change. Like other systems, the potential for entropy or negentropy is present, and thus much depends upon the movements of the actors in the system. And as Sherry Turkle noted recently, an asocial environment is created by computers. Computers, therefore, may serve to implode dialogue.

In order for change to occur in the therapeutic relationship, more than techniques are needed. C. B. Truax (1969) reports that empathy, warmth, and genuineness are the key elements in a helping relationship. Carl Rogers (1969) and Ned Flanders (1970) point out that empathy is particularly central to the helping relationship. Richard Mackey (1985, p.74) summarized the importance of the points made by Truax, Rogers, and Flanders as follows:

> "The most viable resource in clinical work is the self of the therapist—the self as represented in one's biopsychosocial history tempered by professional knowledge, values and skills...The reality that one human being has sought another for assistance suggests that the empathic presence of the latter has a special and potentially profound effect on the outcome of work between them."

Presently, a microcomputer cannot provide the important ingredients of empathy, warmth, genuineness, and authenticity, all of which are key components in successful therapy. No matter how sophisticated the program, these factors have not been built into a computer's repertoire of actions. The ethical dilemma posed by computer technology in clinical practice becomes particularly evident, when client-therapist interaction is recognized to be essential for therapy to occur.

Some studies document that computers produce results similar to or better than trained therapists. The question must be raised: is a catharsis the same as therapy? There is no doubt that clients may find themselves uncomfortable in a therapeutic relationship. Therapeutic dialogue involves social contact that may be difficult. Yet also, social competence involves interpersonal contact. The catharsis may be taking place during computerized therapy may represent nothing more than a technological "fix", designed to secure adequate social functioning. But is coping the same as self-development and growth? Even in the long-run these traits may look similar, while the quality of life in each case may be dramatically different. This is the same objection that is lodged against behaviorists by humanists. None the less, the issue is certainly worth considering. An ethnographic study of computerized therapy may be necessary before the real effects of this style of intervention are understood.

CONCLUSIONS AND IMPLICATIONS

Computer technology is not going to disappear. If anything, the use of computers will become more prevalent. Even with the increasing sophistication of computers, practitioners should be wary about the use of this new technology in clinical practice. A number of concerns have been raised that suggest practitioners should cautiously approach computer technology. These center on the quantitative nature of computer technology and the ways computers may dehumanize the therapeutic relationship.

Presently, clinical social workers employ many treatment strategies that cannot easily be translated into the binary logic of computer technology. Due to the utsiquity of qualities such as empathy, warmth, genuineness, and authenticity, the therapeutic relationship has a qualitative character. Therefore, therapeutic discourse resists computerization. As argued by a number writers, computer technology is so different from the other conventional form of assessment and intervention, the very nature of the therapeutic relationship is transformed to the extent that treatment may be radically altered (Erdman, et. al. 1981). Clinical social workers should explore these changes as computer technology is introduced into clinical practice. Such a critical assessment should help to insure that when computer technology is adopted, these devices complement the interpersonal discourse that is at the core of the treatment process.

REFERENCES

Barnett, G. O. The Computer and Clinical Judgement In M. D.Schwartz, (Ed), *Using Computers In Clinical Practice* (pp.221-224). (New York: The Haworth Press.

Beaumont, J. G. (1982). System Requirements for Interactive Testing, *Man-Machine Studies*, October, 311-320.

Burnham, D. (1980) *The Rise Of The Computer State*. New York: Vintage Books.

Carr, A. C. et al., (1982) Direct Assessment of Depression by Microcomputer, *Computers in Psychiatry/Psychology*, 4, 11-13.

Erdman, H. P. et al., (1981). The Computer Psychiatrist: How Far Have We Come? Where Are We Heading? How Far Dare We Go? *Behavior Research Methods and Instrumentation*, 13, 393-398.

Freud, A. (194). The Widening Scope Of Indicators For Psychoanalysis, *Journal Of The American Psychoanalytic Association*, 2, 607-620.

Flanders, N. A. (1970). *Analyzing Teaching Behaviors*. Reading, Mass: Addison-Wesley Publishing.

Gill, M. M. (1982). *Analysis Of Transference*, Vol. 1 New York: International Universities Press.

Gripton, J. "Computerizing Your Practice," *Practice Digest*, 6, 16-20.

Hall, C. (1983). Psychiatrists' Computer Use Stirs Debate *Wall Street Journal*, December 6.

Hudson, W. W. (1982). *The Clinical Measurement Package: A Field Manual*. Homewood, Illinois: Dorsey Press.

Imre, R. W. (1984). The Nature of Knowledge in Social Work, *Social Work*, 29, 41-45.

Levy, C. S. (1982). *Guide to Ethical Decisions and Actions for Social Service Administrators*. New York: The Haworth Press.

Mackey, R. A. (1985) *Ego Psychology And Clinical Practice*. New York: Gardner Press.

Matarazzo, J. D. (1983). "Computerized Psychological Testing". *Science*, July 22, 221.

Murphy, J. W. and Pardeck, J. T. "Technologically Mediated Therapy: A Critique," *Social Casework*, 67, 605-612.

Pardeck, J. T. and Murphy, J. W. (1986). Microcomputer Technology In Clinical Social Work Practice: Benefits and Problems *Arete*, 11, 35-43.

Reid, G. H. and Gorsuch, R. L. (1984). "Development and Clinical Use of Test-Interpretive Programs on Microcomputers," In M. D. Schwartz, (Ed.), *Using Computers in Clinical Practice* (pp.7-17) New York: The Haworth Press.

Reitman, R. (1984). "The Use of Small Computers in Self-Help Sex Therapy." In M. D. Schwartz, (Ed.), *Using Computers In Clinical Practice*. New York: The Haworth Press (pp. 363-380).

Rogers, C. R. (1969). *Freedom To Learn*. Columbus, Ohio: Charles E. Merrill.

Schinka, J. A. and Smith, R. B. (1984). "The Computer in the Psychotherapist's Office: Present and Future Applications." In M. D. Schwartz (Ed), *Using Computers in Clinical Practice* (pp. 7-17). New York: The Haworth Press.

Skinner H. A. and Allen, B. A. (1983). Does The Computer Make A Difference? Computerized Versus Face-To-Face Versus Self-Report Assessment of Alcohol, Drug, and Tobacco Use, *Journal of Consulting and Clinical Psychology*, 52, 267-275.

Spitzer, R. L. (1983) Psychiatric Diagnosis: Are Clinicians Still Necessary, *Comprehensive Psychiatry* 24, 401-410.

Strong, S. R. and Claiborn, C. D. (1982). *Change Through Interaction: Social Psychological Processes Of Counseling* and *Psychotherapy*. New York: John Wiley and Sons.

Truax, C. B. (1969). "Therapist Empathy, Warmth, and Genuineness, and Patient Personality Change In Group Psychotherapy: A Comparison Between Interaction Unit Measures, Time Sample Measures, and Patient Measures," *Journal of Clinical Psychology*, 71, 1-9.

Weizenbaum, J. (1976). *Computer Power and Human Reason*. San Francisco, CA: W. H. Freeman and Company.

Wolberg, L. R. (1977). *The Technique of Psychotherapy*. New York: Grune and Stratton

6

An Analysis of Critical Concerns in the Use of Computer Technology in Clinical Practice

John W. Murphy, PhD
Associate Professor of Sociology, Department of Sociology, University of Miami

John T. Pardeck, MSW, PhD
Professor and Chair, Department of Social Work, Southeast Missouri State University

Technology is proliferating in every area of society, including clinical practice. Computer programs are now available that conduct in-take interviews, administer, score, and interpret clinical instruments, monitor treatment plans, and engage clients in actual therapeutic discourse (Murphy and Pardeck, 1986a; Pardeck; 1988). Many practitioners believe that these developments will improve the delivery of clinical services. They contend that because this technology performs most activities faster and more accurately than humans, patient care is more effective. Because clinical software packages are unaffected by human judgments, the claim is made that diagnoses and correctives free from error can be provided.

This use of technology in clinical settings, however, has not gone unchallenged (Murphy and Pardeck, 1986a: Murphy and Pardeck, 1986c). One of the most sophisticated critiques of this trend has been formulated by Matarazzo (1986). This paper should be viewed as an attempt to build on his work. Nonetheless, he neglects an area of concern that deserves serious attention. A key shortcoming of his analysis is that he portrays technology to be a tool, which may be used either correctly or incorrectly. His approach overlooks an important finding by researchers in the area of artificial intelligence (AI) that suggests computer technology should not be conceptualized in this manner. Simply put, Matarazzo ignores what Jacques Ellul (1964) calls the "technological ethic". By doing this, the subtle ways in which the logic of data processing may alter clinical practice cannot be fully appreciated.

Modern writers contend that computers do not operate on the basis of technical knowledge alone. What this means is that computers are not value-free, contrary to the view held by many practitioners. In fact, in order for computers to process information effectively, particular theoretical assumptions must be accepted as valid. Taken together, these philosophical principles constitute what writers such as Marvin Minsky and Seymour Papert call the computer "micro-world".

The introduction of this construct into the area of computer studies is quite revolutionary. For example, computers must now be understood to provide their own data selection guidelines. Computers are not merely receptacles into which data are placed, but play an active role in conceptualizing various aspects of social life. Most important, as illustrated by Hubert and Stuart Dreyfus (1986), the computer micro-world is able to create the illusion that computers generate information untrammeled by situational exigencies. Commenting on the GIGO principle, Ashley Montague states that it has come to be misconstrued to mean "garbage in-*gospel* out" (Roszak, 1986, p. 120). Computer-produced knowledge, in other words, is commonly accepted to embody pure reason, unadulterated by interpretation.

The computer micro-world, because it is sustained by judgments that are presumed to be universally acceptable, is able to lull persons into believing that opinion can be separated categorically from fact (Murphy and Pardeck, 1986b). To quote Guattari (1984, p. 114), the process of computerization introduces the "differentiators" necessary to reinforce the usual distinction made between subjectivity and objectivity. This demarche is accomplished by defining key aspects of the clinical milieu in technical terms. As a result, the "technological ethic" becomes integral to clinical activities.

Ellul demonstrates how this ethic enables persons to control practically any process more completely than ever before. Before proceeding, however, what he means by this idea must be clarified. Basic to Ellul's concept is that whenever possible technology should be introduced to formalize a job. Subsequent to translating cognitive operations into technical terms, for example, any task can be organized according to exact calculations. Because the implementation of technical criteria allegedly does not require interpretation, objective or unbiased assessments are deemed possible. Technical competence thus becomes the cornerstone of clinical practice. Yet in order to appreciate how this legerdemain is perpetrated, the computer micro-world must be examined further.

When developing software packages, the assumption is made that persons are "rule-following, symbol-manipulating, rational beings" (Dreyfus and Dreyfus, 1986, p. 132). Evident in this description is the dualistic nature of language. Symbols are manipulated, thus suggesting that they exist independent of human intentions. Therefore, facts are stripped of their interpretive meaning and easily classified. In point of fact, computerization presupposes that symbols represent "context-independent, objective features of the real world" (Dreyfus and Dreyfus, 1986, p. 53). If this were not the case, information could never be introduced into a computer.

Stated otherwise, language must be transformed into a system of "digitalized signs" (Guattari, 1984, p. 87). This occurs when the two elements of the sign/signifier relationship are imagined to be isomorphic. Thus language does nothing more than "point to", "indicate", or "describe" something other than itself (Mitchell, 1986). As Jacques Derrida (1973, p. 138) writes, speech "defers" to factors that are considered to be more fundamental than linguistic acts. Most relevant to this discussion, data are treated as inert objects, or "input", that can be made to conform readily to the logistical demands imposed by computer programs. With this in mind, Jean-Francois Lyotard (1984, p. 86) declares that the appropriate unit of knowledge in the so-called Computer Age is the information "bit". Accordingly, knowledge is transformed into "quantities of information", while data are "externalized" with respect to a knower. This view is shared by Theodore Roszak (1986, pp. 108-134) when he writes that computers deal with idealized knowledge.

Computers can process information only when data are divorced from situational contingencies and, thus, unambiguous. These machines regulate effectively how symbols are used by requiring that data fit exactly into the "conceptual digits" adopted by computer programs to classify input. As described by J. David Bolter (1984, pp. 83-90), each piece of information is assigned an "address space" into which it must be placed. Furthermore, data with uncertain parameters defy this type of classification. And because data are treated in this way, Hubert Dreyfus (1972, pp. 235-255) charges that computerization "disembodies" information, for knowledge is deprived of the interpretive qualities that lend it a human character. Therefore, no-one should be surprised when Margaret Boden (1977, pp. 15-17) argues that computers do not "crunch" numbers, but, more important, define how symbols may be utilized. But how does this change in thinking about computers affect clinical practice?

The remainder of this paper will assess a few of the problems resulting from the technological ethic. Specifically, the purpose of the following discussion is to demonstrate how the computer micro-world may alter significantly the way in which clinical practice is undertaken. Specifically noteworthy is that a thorough study of the ethical problems associated with the use of computer technology by practitioners must address far more than procedural or technical concerns.

Central to the technological ethic is a unique portrayal of social life (Murphy and Pardeck, 1985). Don Ihde, for instance, maintains that computers convey imagery that "deanimates" the clinical setting. He refers to the resulting conception of reality as "instrumental realism", because all phenomena are identified and organized according to the strictures imposed by formal logic and mathematics (Ihde, 1979). Although Matarazzo recognizes that computers unduly objectify data, the rationale he invokes to support this observation is unclear. By introducing the notion of instrumental realism, however, this fault in Matarazzo's argument can be rectified. Simply put, the computer micro-world is *designed* to objectify events, and thus, as Matarazzo notes, clinical evaluations are equated with testing rather than assessment.

Testing in this context refers to the gathering of data through a technical means. Implied is that sentiments corroborated by a so-called objective standard are more valid than subjective expressions. Through standardization and formalization the subjectivity that is assumed to threaten the discovery of truth is controlled. In fact, unless a client's statements are confirmed by a test, most often these claims are dismissed as irrelevant. Testing, therefore, provides access to facts that are available to rational (scientific) inquirers.

Tests produce findings, while assessments are more encompassing and include the element of human sensitivity. Assessments, in other words, are not based solely on technical criteria. However, the presumption that the use of tests can be equated with the generation of high quality data is believed to be entirely justified. When technologically mediated, every facet of a clinical setting is defined in such a way that testing is viewed naturally to produce valid information. This process whereby computerization encodes patients constitutes the social component of the technological ethic. As described by Guattari (1984, pp. 135-143), a patient's behavior is envisaged to be "subjectless action". Actually, what is most problematic about technologically mediated therapy is the tacit suggestion that diagnoses can be objectified without any loss of meaning. Yet the question remains to be answered, what are the ethical consequences of this viewpoint?

1. In any theory of ethics the issue of epistemology must be addressed, for truth provides the foundation of social order. Therapeutic discourse must be based on norms, or facts, that apply to both therapists and patients. Computerization demands that facts be treated as if they are thing-like, as required by the logic of data processing. Those who use computers can manipulate data in an almost unlimited number of ways, yet each piece of information can have only a single identity. In fact, interpretation is thought to interfere with the accurate classification of input. Subjectivity, simply put, is anathema to scientific data collection. The computer micro-world conveys the idea subtly that facts sequestered from interpretation are the most reliable source of knowledge. In this sense, a computer supplies an unambiguous set of rules, sometimes called "effective procedures", that regulate client-therapist interaction.

2. Considering the image of knowledge associated with computerization, the fact that evaluation comes to be synonymous with testing should not be surprising. For facts unmolested by opinion are believed to hold the key to a valid diagnosis. A patient, therefore, must be treated as having traits similar to anyone who has the same malady. Yet, as recognized by Matarazzo, an identical test profile does not necessarily have the same meaning for every client. When diagnoses are guided by

axiomatic principles, however, such a finding suggests the presence of human error. The possibility that a particular symptom may be understood in a variety of ways, depending on cultural or other interpretive factors, is ignored. This is what the Dreyfuses (1986, p. 76) have in mind when they state that expert systems are internally consistent, but oblivious to the world. As a result, each client is approached as a "typical" case.

3. When knowledge is objectified and data collection deanimated, due to the use of formalized methods, judgments are often based on information that may not be relevant. Because computerization idealizes one type of information, while diminishing the importance of others, data derived from technical procedures are assumed to be most germane to making a diagnosis. Moreover, as Kleinmuntz (1984) suggests, reduced reliance on intuitive insight is believed to improve the accuracy of clinical judgments. Yet as diagnostic skill comes to be equated with technical competence, the art of intervention begins to disappear. And when technical standards are not socially paramount, modes of behavioral classification that are technically based are reductionistic. This sort of reductionism is prevalent when so-called "soft" information is treated automatically as ancillary to quantitative data. Such myopia may invalidate altogether the diagnostic process.

4. Giving "calculative rationality" primacy when making a diagnosis tends to engender a particular type of relationship between a client and therapist (Dreyfus and Dreyfus, 1986, pp. 163-167). Furthermore, this style of interaction may not be fruitful, because, using Michel Foucault's (1973, pp. 3-21) terminology, the therapist's gaze is "mathematized". By this he means that clinical discourse is reified. For instance, a client must be approached objectively, for otherwise a clinician's judgments will be sullied by non-empirical elements. Therefore, a patient is assumed to represent a composite of facts, and thus can be examined as simply another "case". As Martin Buber might say, the client and therapist are encouraged to address each other in an "I-it" manner, or stated otherwise, as objects to be manipulated (Murphy, 1983).

Yet how valid can a diagnosis be when a client and therapist to not respect each other? In a now classic statement, Joseph Weizenbaum (1976, p. 270), creator of the interactive program ELIZA, declares that respect is not a technical issue. With this remark he is criticizing those who maintain that therapy can or should be computerized. For without interpersonal sensitivity how can persons help one another? As Buber notes, therapists must confirm their patients during therapy, or mutual understanding will never be achieved. Yet devoid of such intimacy, therapy is nothing more than a means whereby one person coerces another. It is for this reason that contemporary writers, such as Jacques Derrida, Jacques Lacan, and Gilles Deleuze, claim that psychologists and psychiatrists are nowadays effective agents of social control.

Nonetheless, the point of this discussion is to suggest that a computer is not simply a tool, for it is underpinned by specific philosophical assumptions that may shape the clinical setting. The computer micro-world, in other words, contains a social component that is able to dictate the nature of therapeutic discourse. As Matarazzo suggests, this underside of technology may reinforce the objectivity thesis to such an extent that a client's needs are distorted. Yet, most important, is that computerization is dangerous and not necessarily computers.

Accordingly, the overt misuse of computer technology should not necessarily be the focus of ethical concerns. Everyone knows that technology can be used inappropriately. What is mostly overlooked, however, are the subtle ways in which computers can alter therapy. What sort of social imagery is spawned by computerization? For example, how are facts, clients, and the therapeutic relationship conceptualized? Clearly, faulty conceptualization can cause ethical problems.

As should be recognized, the components of therapy are not viewed very positively in terms of the computer micro-world. Clients are presumed to be things, who should be classified in the most efficient manner possible. When this is the case, the thrust of therapy becomes screening and assigning treatment modalities. Little emphasis is placed, in other words, on understanding how clients interpret their actions. After all, the result of this sort of inquiry is considered to be "soft" data. Clinical insight is deemed to be a poor substitute for objective findings.

Most important, the integrity of clients is not violated only by the misuse of technology. Through the correct use of computers clients can be abused. In short, a client can be misclassified, misunderstood, and thus made to conform to standards that have no relevance. Moreover, this misconduct may go unnoticed for a long-time, because computers are believed to be unbiased. How many persons are willing to admit that data are manipulated by computers? Or, maybe more important, how many clients will feel comfortable challenging a computer-based diagnosis? Through the use of computers, therefore, biases may be reinforced. Under the guise of science, erroneous judgments may be made regularly about clients. In a manner of speaking, the abuse of clients may be concealed by computer technology, due to the acceptance of certain implicit assumptions about reality. Actually, every therapist knows that unquestioned assumptions are dangerous to a client. Nonetheless, the assumptions associated with science and computerization are often overlooked. These presuppositions, therefore, operate with impugnity. Clients are thus at risk of being violated by computerization. Certainly this should be a pressing ethical concern. When using computer technology appropriately can become problematic, a whole new dimension of ethics is opened.

The trouble with computerized therapy is that practitioners may begin to think technological refinements are sufficient to improve therapy. Yet this may not be the case, for compassion, support, and understanding are not technical issues. And purged of these elements, how can therapy be effective? Through behavioral modification a client's actions can be altered, yet this sort of change unaccompanied by understanding boarders on manipulation. Do therapists want to be nothing more than agents of social control? Of course not!

Nonetheless, patients and therapists must travel the road of therapy together, in order to avoid transforming the therapeutic encounter into a process of normalization. Client and therapist must approach one another as fellow human beings, rather than as experts who must save clients from themselves. Yet computerization may not foster such symmetry. Ensconced behind a wall of technology, therapists are placed beyond the reach of their clients. As a result, objectivity comes to be equated with impersonality. Yet again, is this kind of insensitivity ethical? Clients may divulge information under this condition, but the therapist is similar to a voyeur. Information is gained without intimacy. In the long run, will this knowledge prove to be useful?

In fine, the use of computers opens a new area of investigation for ethicists and social practitioners. The *proper use* of science and technology *per se* must be the focus of concern, rather than extreme cases malfeasance, life-threatening scenarios, or the distribution of life-saving gadgets. The violence that can occur through the normal operation of computer-based therapy must receive serious attention. This is the new challenge for those who deliver social services.

REFERENCES

Boden, M. (1977). *Artificial Intelligence and Natural Man.* New York: Basic Books.

Bolter, J. D. (1984). *Turing's Man: Western Culture in the Computer Age.* Chapel Hill: University of North Carolina Press.

Derrida, J. (1973). *Speech and Phenomena.* Evanston: Northwestern University Press.

Dreyfus, H. L. (1972). *What Computers Can't Do.* New York: Harper and Row.

Dreyfus, H. L. & Dreyfus, S. E. (1986). *Mind over Machine.* New York: The Free Press.

Ellul, J. (1964). *The Technological Society.* New York: Random House.

Foucault, M. (1973). *The Birth of the Clinic.* New York: Vintage Books.

Guattari, F. (1984). *Molecular Revolution.* New York: Penguin Books.

Ihde, D. (1979). *Technics and Praxis.* Dordrecht: D. Reidel.

Kleinmuntz, B. (1984). The Scientific Study of Clinical Judgments in Psychology and Medicine. *Clinical Psychology Review,* 4, 111-126.

Lyotard, J-F. (1984). *The Postmodern Condition: A Report on Knowledge.* Minneapolis: University of Minnesota Press.

Matarazzo, J. D. (1986). Computerized Clinical Test Interpretations: Unvalidated Plus all Mean and no Sigma. *American Psychologist,* 41, 14-24.

Mitchell, W. J. T. (1986). *Iconology: Image, Text, Ideology.* Chicago: University of Chicago Press.

Murphy, J. W. (1983). *The Social Philosophy of Martin Buber.* Washington, D. C.: University Press of America.

Murphy, J. W. & Pardeck, J. T. (1985). The Technological World-View and the Responsible Use of Computers in the Classroom. *Journal of Education*, 167, 98-108.
Murphy, J. W. & Pardeck, J. T. (1986a). Technology and the Manufacture of Madness: A New Dimension". *The International Journal of Social Psychiatry*, 32, 41-46.
Murphy, J. W. & Pardeck, J. T. (1986b). Computers and Cognitive Development: A Preliminary Statement. *Early Child Development and Care*, 25, 221-230.
Murphy, J. W. & Pardeck, J. T. (1986c). Computerized Clinical Practice: Promises and Shortcomings. *Psychological Reports*, 59, 1099-1113.
Murphy, J. W., Mickunas, A. & Pilotta, J. J. (Eds.). (1986) *The Underside of High-tech.* Westport, CT: Greenwood Press.
Pardeck, J. T. (1988). Microcomputer Technology in Clinical Practice: An Analysis of Ethical Issues. *Journal of Independent Social Work*, 2, 71-81.
Roszak, T.(1986). *The Cult of Information.* New York: Pantheon Books.
Weizenbaum, J. (1976). *Computer Power and Human Reason.* New York: W. H. Freeman.

7

Expert Systems as an Adjunct to Clinical Practice: A Critique

John W. Murphy, PhD
Associate Professor of Sociology, Department of Sociology, University of Miami

John T. Pardeck, MSW, PhD
Professor and Chair, Department of Social Work, Southeast Missouri State University

One product of artificial intelligence (AI) research has been the "expert system". Computer programs have been available for some time that can play checkers, although none of them perform at a very sophisticated level. More elaborate programs such as DENDRAL and MYCIN have been created recently to undertake specific tasks. The purpose of an expert system, simply put, is to replicate the decision making ability exhibited by experts, minus the human error associated with interpretation. In other words, software packages have been developed that allegedly duplicate the cognitive activities vital to decision making, thereby allowing unbiased judgments to be made.

Obviously many routine decisions can be undertaken by a machine, thus reducing personnel costs. After all, computers are undaunted by personal problems and situational exigencies. Advocates of expert systems argue that once the protocol used for decision making are identified, these rules can be built into a software package. Edward Feigenbaum refers to this type of programming as "knowledge engineering" (Dreyfus and Dreyfus, 1986, pp. 101-103). Experts are interviewed to discover the criteria they use when making decisions, and subsequently this information is established as the "knowledge base" of a program. Once this knowledge is codified, a framework is provided that allows a computer to respond to further input in a manner expected from an expert.

All this sounds so simple. As a result of formulating a series of "If...then" statements, computers are given the ability to react intelligently to events. For example, if A is presented, then the computer will respond with B. Translated into the delivery of social services, a diagnosis could hypothetically be rendered in this manner. For every trait A, the remedy B would be prescribed. INTERNIST-1, a program for making diagnoses in internal medicine, operates in this manner.

Furthermore, the DSM-III is based on similar logic. The question that remains, however, is: Do persons make decisions in the mechanistic manner suggested by the typical "If...then" format?

In order to examine properly expert systems, computerization must be understood to represent a mode of conceptualization. This claim becomes evident when examining the operation of an expert system. Specifically, as maintained by Hubert Dreyfus, the belief that computers mimic the functioning of the mind makes sense only if human cognition and computerization are similar. Key assumptions about how the mind is structured and processes information must be accepted as valid. Dreyfus (1979, pp.159-224) refers to these as the biological, psychological, epistemological, and ontological assumptions.

The biological assumption relates to the belief that the mind can be characterized as a network of off/on switches. Mental activity, accordingly, consists of electrical impulses that are correlated with certain stimuli. Presented with a particular stimulus, the mind reacts in an "all or none" fashion that is associated with any "normal" person. Once a stimulus reaches a specific threshold, a switch is triggered and a datum is imprinted on the mind. As a result of this process, knowledge about the world is acquired.

That knowledge can be treated legitimately as "bits" of data, organized according to formal rules, is the basis of the psychological assumption. What this viewpoint suggests is that humans are simply rational, as Herbert Simon (1969, pp.24-25) suggests. In line with what the empiricist Thomas Hobbes contends, reason is heralded to be a form of "reckoning", whereby clearly delineated entities are enumerated. The mind, in a sense, works as a grand calculator. Data with exact parameters are simply classified and tallied. Counting, accordingly, is presumed to be a fundamental cognitive property.

Essential to the epistemological assumption is that knowledge can be formalized, without any appreciable distortion. The aim of formalization is to create absolute rules of reasoning, divorced from quotidian concerns. Usually this belief is manifested in the view that reasoning proceeds according to universal rules of logic. Sometimes this contention is referred to as the "constancy hypothesis". Indigenous to every reasonable person are specific mental categories, along with the connectors that hold them together. Therefore, every mind is accompanied by a similar data base, thus establishing a universal frame of reference for judging whether or not an action makes sense.

According to the ontological assumption, knowledge consists of "discrete, explicit, and determinate" data (Dreyfus, 1979, p. 206). Most important at this juncture is that knowledge is thought to be purely empirical. Facts, for instance, are associated with obtrusive features, thus enabling data to be easily categorized. The symbolic or interpretive side of knowledge is overlooked, simply because this source of information is cited to be subjective and unreliable.

Because expert systems are supposed to act like human experts, the mind and a computer are presumed to be alike. Of course, if cognition is understood to operate similar to a machine, then programming a computer to "think" is at least possible. Although the relationship between knowledge and the mind can be conceived in a causal manner, this imagery is quite restrictive. For example, clarity and procedural rigor are identified as sufficient for generating judgments that have social utility. Yet when the mind is imagined to be equivalent to a physical system, goodness of fit between its parts is the focus of attention. For essential to a smooth running machine is that its components mesh tightly together.

Establishing an adequate knowledge base, therefore, is basic to developing an expert system. Minsky and Papert (1973), for instance, state that this body of information consists of "structural primitives" or "primitive symbols". What they mean is that boundaries must be outlined with respect to knowledge commonly accepted, for example, about facts, relationships, priorities, and purposes. Accordingly, expert systems resemble "analytical engines" once this task is accomplished. The responses elicited by input are regulated by the "stock of knowledge" presupposed by a program, rather than emotional or interpretive issues. For this reason, precise input generates output devoid of ambiguity.

Stated in another way, according to Roger Schank and Robert Abelson (1977, pp.36-68), expert systems are organized around "scripts", which are believed to contain all the information necessary for a person to make an informed judgment. "Prototypical" elements that are pivotal to identifying a specific phenomenon are specified. These factors, accordingly, delimit the range of rational inquiry. As input is verified against these variables, a stereotypical response follows. If a piece of information happens to fit into the analytical scheme that is provided, reason appears to be exhibited by a computer. As described by Terry Winograd (1972, pp. 23-28), expert systems are made operational through a style of programming that isolates a "mini-world", which is assumed to be generalizable to everyday life. Due to such model building, expert systems are touted to behave like experts.

Yet is the model of the mind inaugurated by expert systems technology adequate? In other words, do expert systems and human cognition operate in an identical manner? If isomorphism actually existed between these two phenomena, the mind could be structured according to functionalist principles. Indeed, cognition could be divided neatly into a variety of mental activities, with each one assigned a particular task to perform. Each component of the mind, moreover, could be understood as activated by a single stimulus found in the environment. For if a stimulus is unencumbered by extraneous factors and the mind is not damaged, data can be easily classified and thus properly recorded. Conceived in this manner, the mind is a "data processor" and requires only clear information channels in order to regulate knowledge. "Noise", or unwanted insight, must be purged from the transmission of information. Hence the mind becomes a means for accepting input, channeling throughput, and generating output.

Considering this portrayal of the mind, no-one should be surprised that expert systems are believed to enhance decision making (Dreyfus and Dreyfus, 1986, pp. 101-121). According to functionalists, reason is equated with a person's ability to analyze input effectively and efficiently. Because an expert system can accommodate a vast amount of data, due to the formalization of information, the power of the mind can be increased. Improved precision and the availability of a large amount of information are thought to facilitate rational action, for data that the mind could not otherwise handle can be introduced into a deliberation process. Intelligence, in this sense, is nothing but the ability to manage facts, while rationality is predicated on the size of a person's data base.

Cognitive activity consists of the process whereby the mind follows the instructions provided to assess input. Some modern writers label this a "turn key" approach to cognition (Davis, 1986, p. xii). Simply described, cognition occurs when the causal relationship between input and output is undisturbed. Yet, the question must be asked, is reason simply the ability to process input? Does the mind respond to stimuli, based on the "control knowledge" built into an abstract model of intelligence? (Dreyfus, 1979, pp. 29-31). Is it safe to assume that clear information channels will insure that input produces a socially acceptable behavioral response?

Rational behavior is usually identified to have several important characteristics. First, persons who are rational are able to survey an array of data and correctly classify these items. Second, the categorization of input is accomplished in terms of probability statements that reflect accurately the criteria assumed to differentiate reality from illusion. And third, responses to input fall within an acceptable range of behavior, thereby enabling persons to anticipate each other's actions. Accordingly, facts are assumed to be empirical, objective, and readily accessible to anyone who can approach the world without bias. Clearly if access to a large amount of explicitly defined knowledge is essential to making reliable decisions, an expert system will assist clinicians and other social service workers with their jobs. But, as will be discussed later, Winograd (1973, observes that this portrayal of understanding and reason is quite "brittle", or, in other words, narrow and socially insensitive. Yet if persons are merely rational as claimed by Herbert Simon, in that they simply evaluate input and draw conclusions based on this data, then expert systems can be safely assumed to aid decision makers.

A very logical dialogue can be established between a doctor and a computer, for example, through the use of PIP (Present Illness Program) (Pauker, Gorry, Kassirer, and Schwartz, 1984). A young man who has massive pedal edema (a swollen foot) consults a physician. After examining this patient, the doctor consults PIP in the following manner:

1A is pedal edema, which is massive
  1. for days
  2. for weeks
  3. for months
  4. for years (answer)

1B is it,
  1. first time
  2. infrequent
  3. occasional
  4. frequently

1C is it,
  1. without temporal-pattern
  2. worse in morning
  3. worse in evening (answer)

1D is it,
  1. symmetrical
  2. asymmetrical (answer)

1E is it,
  1. pitting
  2. non-pitting (answer)

This type of questioning continues until a full range of social factors and other physical symptoms are identified. Following the completion of the question-answer series, a diagnosis is rendered. As the answers given to questions begin to distinguish one disease from another, a clear and concise etiology is established. Accordingly, a probability statement is generated pertaining to the likelihood that a particular set of symptoms "fits" into a well established syndrome.

MYCIN was designed originally to provide advice about diagnosing and offering proper therapy for infectious diseases, particularly infections of the blood (Dreyfus, 1979, p. 28). A conclusion is reached as a result of studying a variety of the rules that are outlined, such as number eighty-five.

If:
  1. The site of the culture is blood, and
  2. The gram stain of the organism is gramming, and
  3. The morphology of the organism is rod, and
  4. The patient is a compromised host.

Then:
  There is suggestive evidence (.6) that the identity of the organism is pseudomonas-aeruginosa.

A similar format is central to the Diagnostic Interview Schedule (DIS), which can be used to identify psychiatric disorders (Comings, 1984). Information about a problem is obtained through what is sometimes referred to as a "flow chart" methodology. The following prob routine is useful to determine whether or not a "yes" answer means that symptoms are caused by drugs, alcohol, or an incident, such as a physical injury.

Question: "Have you ever had prolong periods when you felt depressed"?

NO: (routine ends)

YES: (Go to next question(s))

Question: "Did you tell any other professional about (Sx)"?

Question: "Did you take medication for (Sx) more than once"?

Question: "Did (Sx) interfere with you life or activities a lot"?

ALL NO:

FIRST YES: (Ask following questions)

Question: "Was (Sx) the result of a physical illness or injury"?

YES: (Go to A in box D)

NO: (Go to No. 3)

Question: "Was (x) always the result of a physical illness or injury (Such as:..............)

YES: Record all

NO: (proceed)

Again, this procedure for charting responses to probe questions allegedly facilitates rational decision making. Because this approach to interrogating a client is precise and methodical, a comprehensive medical or psychological record is thought to be created.

In each of these examples, issues are raised about phenomena that are never seriously questioned. A particular illness, for instance, is presented, along with a list of symptoms and a repertoire of appropriate treatments. Merely by following a clearly delineated set of instructions a diagnosis can be rendered. In a manner of speaking, a diagnosis is the result of identifying input, processing throughput, and producing output. To use behaviorist language, thinking is the activity whereby stimuli and responses are united. When cognition becomes this mechanical, however, the art of making a diagnosis may atrophy, as noted by writers as disparate as

Thorstein Veblen (1964) and Ivan Illich (1976). The reason for this is quite simple: logic is gradually substituted for reasoning and learning. Suggested by this caveat is that reason is not exhausted by formal logic. Restricting cognition in this way, however, may be very problematic.

Once certain principles are accepted as universally valid, making a diagnosis consists of applying a few axioms to individual cases. Such a procedure is thought to increase a practitioner's credibility. Consistent with what Ellul understands to be the "technological imperative" at the basis of Western societies, the human element is removed as much as possible from making a diagnosis. Cognitive operations, simply put, are defined in technical terms. And because techniques are touted to be devoid of interpretation, bias is ostensibly removed from clinical decisions. No wonder Peter Berger (1973, pp.33-35) and his colleagues claim that the centerpiece of modern technology is "emotional management". When diagnostic protocol are transformed into a body of techniques, practitioners can be easily convinced that clinical practices are severed from the values that are ubiquitous to everyday life. After all, technology is applied science, and traditionally science is assumed to be value-free.

As documented by Michel Foucault (1975), clinicians have tried continuously to create the impression that their judgments are objective and scientific. Keeping this idea in mind, is there any better way to bolster clinical practice than by computerizing the collection of patient-related data? As a result of equating precision with accuracy, the information generated through the use of a computer is thought to be very reliable. Because this technology is unaffected by situational factors, judgments are not believed to be capricious. Actually, diagnoses are presumed to be free of interpretation, because a "logic tree" dictates the format of a clinical interview. Further, underpinning this entire enterprise is the belief that if the mind were not clouded by emotional issues, clinicians could act regularly in a rational manner, similar to a computer.

There is little doubt about the precision of the calculations made by a computer, but are they accurate? Do the judgments outlined by a computer program have any *social* significance? Critics of computerized clinical evaluation systems argue that the knowledge base of this technology is too abstract. Stated simply, the knowledge invoked to substantiate decisions is accumulated *without learning* (Dennett, 1984). In other words, the data bank that is associated with expert systems is organized in a vacuum. The ability to deduce a course of action, or treatment, from higher-order principles is thought to be indicative of rationality. Yet is following the logic prescribed by an algorithm the same as learning?

The cognitive practices indigenous to formal logic are pristine, or divorced from intervening variables. Once a set of assumptions is accepted as legitimate, all practitioners have to do is to perform a few simple, yet rigorous, procedures in order to be viewed as competent. Yet is this the way learning proceeds? The early Greeks stated that learning begins with "wonder", while today most educators would agree that tolerance of ambiguity is central to becoming an educated person. Stated differently, learning does not simply involve the application of abstract principles to explain particular events. Instead, education begins when persons question ideas that were previously accepted, recognize that social norms are not universal, and understand that truth cannot be divorced from historical conditions. In other words, education liberates persons from dogmatism. Explanatory principles, accordingly, should not be utilized in a mechanistic or unreflective manner.

Hubert and Stuart Dreyfus (1986, pp. 16-51), as part of their overall critique of AI, maintain that decision making progresses through a variety of stages, ranging from "novice" to "expert". Moreover, they contend that expert systems operate at an elementary level. A novice classifies events in a "context-free" manner, based solely on their empirical traits. As the Dreyfuses illustrate, the letter "E" is recognized because it has vertical and horizonal lines that are arranged in a unique pattern. Beginners focus primarily on following specific rules, regardless of the situation in which a task is initiated. The reason for this narrowness of vision is quite simple: A novice does not yet have a global understanding of his or her job, and thus has no alternative but to solve a problem by adhering to a step-by-step format.

The expert, on the other hand, does not make similar tasks undertaken in different contexts conform to a single *modus operandi*. Rather, experts are able to assess each situation separately, recognize how events are both different and similar, and generate provisional rules about how a "typical" case should be handled. Instead of assuming a reductionistic view, an expert analyzes events holistically, and thus combines a variety of disparate experiences when formulating an opinion. An expert knows when rules should and should not be applied, in addition to when guidelines should be expanded in order to address new findings. Simply put, acquiring an appreciation of the contextual nature of facts is an essential part of becoming an expert.

In terms of the definition proffered by the Dreyfuses, computers can never achieve the status of an expert. Computers operate on the basis of a self-contained context, thereby obscuring situationally relevant factors, while experts do not. Experts are reflexive, aware of contextual limitations, and able to synthesize what at first may appear to be divergent ideas. In this respect, experts do not rely on well-worn formulas, but make use of whatever knowledge is available or necessary to solve a problem. As opposed to detached observers, experts strive to gain insight into the knowledge they acquire. Accordingly, they act rationally, in that social decorum is not violated. Emphasis, in other words, is placed on the interpretive or contextual character of data.

Rather than "technical competence", experts place "communicative competence" at the core of rational behavior (Habermas, 1970). Persons interact rationally or competently when they take into account the assumptions each other makes about reality. Rational behavior, as suggested by the Dreyfuses, is in tune with the expectations persons have about social regulations. Yet, the question must be asked, why is the Dreyfuses' definition relevant to clinicians and other practitioners? Succinctly stated, clinicians must respond directly to their clients, rather than decipher their behavior with respect to rarefied theories and models. In fact, Foucault contends that merely categorizing patients according to an abstract scheme is immoral, because they are treated as objects to be manipulated. As opposed to therapists, those who make behavior conform to a "model man" are simply agents of social control.

Given the intimate nature of a therapeutic encounter, the relevance of expert systems for facilitating rational clinical decision making must be questioned. That is, does the mind function simply in a associationist manner? Obviously this is not the case, for cognition consists of far more than drawing conclusions on the basis axioms that are believed to be unquestioningly valid! Most important, the mind does not simply classify events, but additionally *interprets* whatever is known. Rather than a conduit for knowledge, the mind gives meaning to the information that it processes. The mind, in this sense, is context-bound.

Due to this crucial difference between the mind and a computer, expert systems may not be assumed automatically to improve clinical judgments. Because knowledge is conceptualized in a very restrictive way by computer programs, the data that are produced may prove to be useless. Enamored of technique, however, practitioners may not recognize that precision and accuracy are not synonymous. Actually, rational decision making may be subverted as a result of confusing these two ideas. In lieu of what the Dreyfuses have to say about the social nature of rationality, decision making is improved only by becoming increasingly concrete or socially sensitive. This is certainly true when a clinician attempts to evaluate a client's demeanor. The question remains: How can computers be both rigorous and generate socially relevant data? This concern must be addressed by those who want to use computers for clinical purposes. For as many modern writers show, a client's "world" must be understood before therapy can be successful. Yet the knowledge base of an expert system may not contain the logic employed by clients to make decisions. Accordingly, a diagnosis may be precise but violate a patient's integrity. How can such insensitivity be considered therapeutic?

Expert systems operate on the basis of what Papert (1980) calls "powerful ideas". Explicit definitions, logistical rigor, logic, and error identification are central to the functioning of these devices. Yet are these factors sufficient to guarantee that decisions are relevant? Critics of expert systems say no. Inadvertently dismissed as unimportant is the idea that the mind does not merely respond to events. Nonetheless, the mind does not simply respond to reality. As noted by postmodernists, through conceptual activities reality is shaped. The acceptance of particular assumptions serves to differentiate reality from illusion.

This means that persons are not rational actors, as defined by Simon. The most fundamental cognitive function is not classifying events. Primordial are the mental acts that supply cognitive categories with their significance. Hence essential to rational behavior are the judgments that establish the framework used for distinguishing reason from irrationality. Cognitive categories supply the parameters for outlining the rules of logic. Decision making, therefore, is more existential than logical.

What does this conclusion mean for social practitioners (Lyotard, 1984)? Specifically important, their decision making will not likely be enhanced as result of procedural refinements, for judgments do not have a technical basis. Focusing on procedural issues, accordingly, will not yield positive results. Instead, emphasis should be placed on the contextual character of decisions. Decisions, stated simply, are context-bound. The values, beliefs, and commitments that are operating in a setting must be understood, before proper decisions can be made.

In view of the work undertaken by postmodernists, decision making will be improved only if practitioners become more reflective. Value-freedom and technical precision are not correctives for faulty decisions. Although improved techniques may make the acquisition of knowledge more precise, the resulting information may be irrelevant because its social context is ignored. In order to avoid this travesty, computerization must be placed in the service of interpretation. In fact, this is the thrust of reflexivity.

By remembering a few points, reflexivity can become a prominent theme in development of expert systems. First, technological rationality must no longer be provided with a seignorial status. This form of reason should not be treated as epitomizing rationality, but just another cognitive style. As a result of this reformulation, the knowledge associated with computers cannot be viewed automatically as objective and, thus, socially important.

Second, the logic utilized by expert systems should not assumed to be universal, simply because the claim is made that it is standardized. Because computer logic is recognized to be sustained by a set of reality assumptions that interpret data, information is not only garnered, stored, and processed by computers, but, more important, shaped by the logic of computerization. This understanding alerts persons to the limited validity of any style of knowledge, including that associated with expert systems.

Third, computers must be understood to produce reliable knowledge only if the conceptual digits used to categorize data reflect the cognitive structures that persons employ to organize their everyday lives. In this sense, the logic of data processing must interpret facts in a manner similar to the human action that is being classified. The findings engendered through computerization, therefore, will be socially sensitive, since human cognition and not technological rationality specifies the significance of data.

And fourth, all of the information generated through technology must be verified against its social context. Only in this way can the users of expert systems be sure that they are interpreting a setting, for example, in a manner similar to its inhabitants. This maneuver demonstrates that mutual confirmation among persons is necessary for them to reach a common understanding, and not simply procedural standardization. For social competence is based on interpersonal discourse that cannot be explained in terms of technical skills. Logic is not technical but social.

Social practitioners make decisions about persons, rather than objects. These judgments will be accurate only when they are interpersonally corroborated. Building this sort of rapport, accordingly, is an interpersonal and not a technological issue. What this means is that expert systems must be attuned to the social character of decision making, before these machines will have appreciable utility. Made *in vacuo,* in other words, decisions are speculative and likely irrelevant. Put in the service of interpretation or cognition, however, the chances are improved that expert systems will generate valuable information.

REFERENCES

Berger, P. L., Berger, B., and Kellner, H. (1973). *The Homeless Mind.* New York: Random House.

Comings, D. E. (1984). A Computerized Diagnostic Interview Schedule (DIS) for Psychiatric Disorders. In M. D. Schwartz (Ed.), *Using Computers in Clinical Practice* (pp. 195-203). New York: The Haworth Press.

Davis, D. (1986). *Managing Technological Innovation.* San Francisco: Jossey-Bass.

Dennett, D. (1984). "Cognitive Wheels: The Frame Problem of AI". In C. Hookway (Ed.), *Minds, Machines, and Evolution* (pp. 129-151). Cambridge: Cambridge University Press.

Dreyfus, H. L. (1979). *What Computers Can't Do.* New York: Harper and Row.

Dreyfus, H. L. and Dreyfus, S. E. (1986). *Mind over Machine.* New York: The Free Press.

Ellul, J. (1964). *The Technological Society.* New York: Random House.

Foucault, M. (1975). *The Birth of the Clinic.* New York: Vintage Books.

Habermas, J. (1970). "Towards a Theory of Communicative Competence". In H. P. Dreitzel (Ed). *Recent Sociology,* No. 2 (pp. 115-148). New York: Macmillan.

Illich, I. (1976). *Limits to Medicine.* New York: Penguin Books.

Lyotard, J. F. (1984). *The Postmodern Condition: A Report on Knowledge.* Minneapolis: University of Minnesota Press.

Minsky, M. and Papert, S. (1973). *Artificial Intelligence.* Condon Lectures, Oregon State of Higher Education, Eugene, Oregon.

Papert, S. (1980) *Mindstorms: Children, Computers, and Powerful ideas.* New York: Basic Books.

Pauker, S. G., Gorry, A. G., Kassirer, J. P., and Schwartz, W. B. (1984). Towards the Simulation of Clinical Cognition: Taking a Present Illness by Computer. In W. J. Clancy and E. A. Shortliffe (Eds.), *Readings in Medical Artificial Intelligence* (pp. 131-159). Reading, MA: Addison-Wesley.

Schank, R. and Abelson, R. (1977). *Scripts, Plans, Goals, and Understanding,* Hillsdale, NJ: Lawrence Erlbaum Associates.

Simon, H. A. (1969). *The Sciences of the Artificial.* Cambridge, MA: MIT Press.

Winograd, T. (1972). *Understanding Natural Language.* New York: Academic Press.

Winograd, T. (1973). A Procedural Model of Language Understanding. In R. C. Schank and K. M. Colby (Eds.), *Computer Models of Thought and Language* (pp. 152-186). San Francisco: W. H. Freeman Co.
Veblen, T. (1964). *The Instinct of Workmanship.* New York: Norton

8

Adapting Technology to Human Service Agencies:

The Experience of One Midwest Agency

Michael J. Kelly, Ph.D.
Associate Professor, School of Social Work, 733 Clark Hall, University of Missouri-Columbia, Columbia, Missouri 65201

Howard Jacob Karger, Ph.D.
Associate Professor, Director of Doctoral Education, School of Social Work, Louisiana State University

Social workers have traditionally resisted the introduction of computers into the workplace. Historically, large social agencies began computerizing in the mid-1960s, with most of these agencies using computer technology for indirect services. Gradually, computerization expanded to many direct service activities. Data that were never before available were now regularly utilized. The advent of the terminal-expanded computer usage to the smallest agencies. The greatest change occurred, however, with the introduction in the early 1970s of the micro or personal computer. Sought by even the smallest agencies, these low priced computers are now advancing the revolution in technological applications.

As in all revolutions, the people involved are at times dismayed and delighted. The proponents of computers, particularly micros, proclaim that these machines will have a positive effect on social service agencies. In particular, the working relations of staff, service delivery , and individual freedom and productivity will all improve. Opponents, on the other hand, see computers as replacing human judgement. Specifically, efficiency will be valued over compassion and concern as the human being is subordinated to new mechanical masters.

This chapter discusses these differing points of view, in terms of how they were realized in a social agency which adopted microcomputer technology. Opposing points of view are illustrated by discussing whether computers are tools for the liberation of human expression, or methods for oppressing the very human qualities for which social services are noted.

THE LITERATURE ON MICROCOMPUTERS

The literature concerned with mainframe computers, microcomputers, and computer programs in social welfare and human service settings is growing. Specialized journals, such as *Computers in the Human Service* and *Computers in Psychiatry/Psychology* provide a forum for the expression of a wide variety of computer applications, reviews of software programs, and the discussion of controversial issues. The current literature seems to fall into three major categories.

First, the largest amount of journal space is devoted to computer (both mainframe and micro) applications, which use either specially developed software or commercial "off-the-shelf" programs. This branch of the literature shows an ever-expanding set of experiments and activities, in which the computer is used to aid workers, particularly clinical workers, in their job performance and client activities. Management applications, such as budgeting and word processing, are found less often in the literature. This is likely due to the availability of the large amount of literature on management applications available in business journals and computer magazines. Case studies tend to report on successful applications, on didactic "how to" guides for buying and using equipment, and on programs in which computers play a role in administration activities or as instruments of research. This includes analyses of clinical or quantitative data, education of staff, clients, or consumers, and the acquisition of information by staff or clients.

The second major area encompasses reports and evaluations of software. Journal space is allotted in the specialized human service computer journals to exhaustive evaluations of the software applications developed for the practitioners. Another source, often overlooked, is the "literature" available from newsletters and computer bulletin boards. This less formal source supplies a great deal of the information on applications shared by users.

The final area is allotted to all other discussions of computerization, technology, and criticism. This area is less developed and contains a paucity of empirical literature devoted to the impact of computer technology on workers, clients, and social service administration. There are few studies reported on the effects of computerization, and the helpfulness of this research is largely an article of faith. Critical analyses of user reactions are all but non-existent.

Literature on this latter issue, the focus of this chapter, is often found outside the social service field. Indeed, the literature on artificial intelligence and the effort to make machines that can think in ways similar to humans is typically found in such discussions. Joseph Weizenbaum's *Computer Power and Human Reason* or Herbert Dreyfus's *What Computers Can't Do* are representative of deeply critical works on computerization. Nevertheless, there remains a need for a critical analysis of the role computers play in the human services, and the reaction of human service professionals to this technology.

IMPLEMENTATION

For any organization that relies on secretaries using electric typewriters, case records filled out by hand, or dictation and hand filing, the transition to microcomputers presents problems. These transition-based problems can be viewed as consequence of using microcomputer technology. Consequently, social agencies making the transition are experiencing the pain associated with innovation.

Innovation studies have shown that there is usually one person (or a few) who seeks new methods, ideas, and techniques. These "gatekeepers" bring in new ideas and provide the initial support for innovations. Similarly, some persons eagerly await new ideas, while another group of workers adjusts after a new technique is established and a third resists innovation altogether. These groups are called early, middle, and late adopters. Keeping in mind that new ways of doing things are not easily accepted, the experience of one organization illustrates the nature of the problems associated with adopting microcomputers.

The extension program of the University of Missouri-Columbia, School of Social Work, has been helping agencies adopt microcomputer technology for several years and has produced a planning guide. Extension philosophy suggests that the best strategy for adopting new technology is: (1) involve staff at all levels, (2) study the agency's microcomputer needs, (3) determine available options, (4) get estimates on equipment and program software, and (5) carefully review what will be altered and how and when these changes will be made. In other words, plan rationally and adequately prepare the staff for the change.

Agencies should purchase microcomputers, monitors, disk drives or other storage devices, printers, connection cables, switches, and all other necessary equipment at one time from a reliable supplier. A reliable supplier will repair or replace defective parts, install the system and insure that all the parts work together, train the staff in the use of the system, and consult on problems. However, this situation is ideal and rarely found in small and middle-sized social agencies.

The experience of one organization provides a common example of how the process can work. The Midwest Agency (MA) began its journey into microcomputer technology using an Apple II (purchased in 1980 for a staff member who wanted to do research). At the time, this was a bold step forward. Later, another staff member prepared a large document using a primitive word-processing program, and non-researchers began to see the advantages of using microcomputers for writing tasks. Two more Apples were purchased, this time the Apple II+ model. By 1983, the acceptance of the microcomputer in business assured the growth of new markets and spawned an explosion in computer literacy. Responding to this impetus, the agency decided to spend some of its limited budget on more micros. The move was now made to IBM's new PC model, which is widely touted to be a legitimate management tool.

Purchased primarily because of its word-processing capability, the new IBM computers were turned over to the secretaries who were then provided with an inexpensive word-processing program, and instructed to quickly learn the system. The early adopters were miffed that the new machines were to be used primarily as typewriters, and were angered when the next round of purchases went to program coordinators and directors. Some early adopters purchased personal machines and programs, to which they developed an almost religious devotion.

Another group disturbed by the microcomputer revolution were those people who had used mainframe computers. Most thought that one centrally placed computer was all that was needed. This group reluctantly accepted micros only when they were shown that these machines could act as terminals for mainframe applications. A final group who remained steadfast in their opposition was comprised mostly of direct service practitioners, who saw little advantage in the use of microcomputers. Moreover, this group believed that introducing microcomputers would mechanize their work and reduce its human dimensions.

Equipment and software went through dramatic changes as a multitude of new products were introduced. Moreover, prices began to fall—particularly on hardware—as several companies bitterly fought to dominate the micro market. In addition, new types of printers, different disk storage formats, hundreds of new programs, and new forms of computer/printer sharing devices came on the market. The agency was now faced with a myriad of technical choices, rapidly changing prices, and pressure from staff persons. Part of the staff wanted to see the adoption of their favorite equipment and software, yet others simply wanted micros and were willing to forestall other purchases. The mainframe oriented group wanted one machine, and the resisters remained opposed to all computers.

All of these choices were further complicated by the haphazard method of introducing computers, as well as unforseen consequences. Among the latter were changes in the role of support people, the need for new staff specializations, and problems with information control. Secretaries who had formerly typed for the professional staff now found themselves responsible for the composition of documents, the entry and maintenance of sophisticated client and budget information, the maintenance and submission of required reports, and the education of professional staff about basic computer questions.

In a similar way, new roles surfaced. The complicated problems associated with keeping the equipment running and integrated, resulted in a staff person assuming the role of the "in house" computer expert. Moreover, this position became more powerful once information became more valuable.

Finally, with more staff able to do reports and fiscal analysis—and easily copy files—more information reached more of the staff. A great deal of information, formerly maintained only by the chief administrator, came into the hands of practitioners. Also, workers produced documents and maintained electronic copies, often not adding these items to the central files. This phenomenon resulted in individual banks of information not controlled by the agency.

Along the way, the administration was faced with questions related to replacement and repair, the incompatibility of equipment among different versions and makes of computers, different types of interfaces, a plethora of programs, and a growing number of outputs. For example, difficult choices had to be made between repairing older equipment or replacing equipment with new but incompatible computers. Staff members frequently suggested that the agency should become standardized, in order to limit the number of options. However, standardization was very often opposed. Coalitions were formed around certain options, sometimes bringing together staff members who were ideologically opposed in other areas. Staff debates were frequent and sometimes heated, often complicated by questions of status and the distribution of rewards. This laissez-faire method of introduction made the position of the administrator and computer personnel both difficult and controversial.

Although the actual experience was far from the ideal, illustrated is the more common experience of social agencies—indeed, of most organizations—in purchasing and using microcomputers. This experience forms the basis of the following analysis.

TECHNOLOGY AS A FORCE FOR OPPRESSION

The adoption of microcomputer technology aroused the ire of some workers. Along with many other human service providers, they felt that computers (i.e., the organizational reverence for computers and the "culture" of computer ideas) caused the oppression of human and individual ideals. For many human service professionals, centralization and bureaucratization, over-specialization, machine reviews of performance, lack of worker control, and the reduction of human interaction were hazards inherent to computer use.

For example, Joseph Weizenbaum, a programmer interested in computers as aides to human thinking, developed ELIZA, a program which simulated the dialogue of a Rogerian therapist. Dismayed by the openness with which people treated a simple program, he abandoned further programing and wrote a major critique of computerization (Johnson, 1986: 55-56).

Although not articulated in the same way, Weizenbaum's fears were shared by some Midwest Agency social workers who felt that machines mimicking human interaction would bring about the rejection of humanism in favor of efficient machine-based dialogue. Moreover, they were concerned with the confidentiality of electronic data and the centralization of information, particularly in the hands of a few specialists. These humanists were also offended by the reduction of complex human interactions into simple categories. Lastly, the critics were concerned that technology would eliminate entry level, low-status jobs.

Some fears were based on experiences with large computers. From 1950 until the 1980s, computers in organizations were primarily mainframe types. These million dollar installations occupied preferred quarters, were tended by white coated specialists with enormous influence in organizational matters, and required that work be organized around the capabilities and specifications of the machine. Electronic Data processing (EDP) and management information systems (MIS) demanded specially coded data from workers, in order to produce reports for senior managers on worker efficiency. Information was specialized, centralized, coded, and secret.

Only in the rarest instances was output designed to help the worker or the client. When information was needed, workers had to ask specialists who spoke a difficult technical language. New technology, as is required for direct data entry, was chosen by specialists who directed how and when it was to be used. Social service workers were rarely asked about their data needs. Workers received "error reports" when mistakes were made, but were rarely "tickled" about cases needing review. In addition, they were made to write in a manner required for machines reading and, in return, reports were intelligible only to technicians.

The philosophy accompanied the use of a mainframe was based on uniformity, control, centralization, and specialization. This extended to the terminals, which were appended to mainframes to control hundreds of "work stations." In the largest social service agencies, hundreds of workers spent all day entering and reviewing data on VDTs (video display terminals). This caused concern among professionals that the electromagnetic radiation from VDTs might affect the health of workers, especially pregnant women. Eye strain, back problems, and hand cramps were added concerns. Although extensively studied, the problems remain unresolved. For some critics, technology has failed clearly to address the needs of workers.

The industrial revolution introduced the tyranny of the self-paced machine, a situation reenacted in automated work reviews. Reviewed by computer programs, a worker's every mistake, miscue, or pause is noted and recorded. These records are used to grade work effort and speed, in addition to creating production schedules which lead to standards that can be easily changed and "piece rate" payment systems.

Related to the automated review is the "homework" concept. Connected by a modem to the host mainframe, workers perform data processing tasks from home. Organizations use homework to employ single parents with small children, the physically handicapped, and others who cannot work outside their homes. The organization saves on buildings, parking, and full-time employee benefits, and has a work force that can be easily idled when demand is low. These unorganized employees work alone—usually on a "piece work" basis—and thus can be easily exploited. Computers have also affected the numbers and types of employment available. Many basic assembly and fabrication plants have become automated, thereby reducing the demand for blue collar workers.

These were some of the fears of the Midwest Agency staff. Computers, and the power given to them by people, represent a formidable force that can oppress workers and clients.

TECHNOLOGY AS A FORCE FOR LIBERATION

The Midwest Agency's experience with computer technology was based on the microcomputer. Microcomputers represent a dramatic challenge to the mainframe philosophy of centralization and control. These devices are personal tools, which can provide individuals with a satisfying computer environment. In this way, micros minimize the centralization and control of information identified with oppression. Indeed, they provide a mechanism for enhancing the expression of creativity on the part of workers and clients. According to this scenario, microcomputer technology can encourage liberation.

The role of microcomputers as agents of liberation is evidenced by the fact that the directors of some MIS and EDP departments in social agencies tried to prohibit their introduction. These departments knew that decentralizing information technology would threaten their control. The great threat for these departments lay in having individuals produce and use their own information, a process which eroded the power base long enjoyed by MIS and EDP departments. In the end, power became more evenly distributed, once information was disseminated throughout the agency.

The Midwest Agency's experience shows the potentially liberating influence of microcomputer technology. First, micro's were introduced initially at the request of workers. First one person, and then a small group sought micros and decided what information would be collected and how these data should be used. It was as if managers had given their permission for these individuals to collect and utilize data as they please. This is rare, even in most professional organizations. For these early users, the micro represented a democratic technology which they were allowed to master.

The middle adopters followed the first group in embracing micros, and encouraged the agency to make the investment needed to purchase this technology. Management responded by allocating computers for administrative tasks, a decision which helped some, but not all, middle adopters. An unexpected, but liberating force was again generated. New alliances, new relationships, and a new respect for the interconnectedness of professional and supportive staff emerged. A users group—a kind of self-help computer club—emerged between the support staff and professionals. After knowing a lot about machine use, support staff members were able to initiate meaningful interaction with professionals. This nascent communication led to the solution of a number of working problems.

Support and professional staff found new ways to coordinate their efforts and, because of better communication and improved inter-staff understanding, clients received higher quality services. On their own, support staff began to analyze operations and outcomes, and pointed out new ways to organize the flow of work and improve services. For example, as productivity and budget information became easily stored on computer disks, workers who formerly lacked access to this information could now study and propose new administrative proposals. The widespread use of microcomputers also reduced managerial control over information, which depended on the centralized storage of data. Because of staff interests and professional concerns agencies experienced a new openness, as worker input increased and new methods for handling fiscal resources were explored.

Workers who had readily adapted to the new technology found their work patterns and outcomes positively affected. Professionals, who composed notes by hand and were dependent on typists, were reluctant to consume more time by redrafting. With word processors, they could redraft a psycho-social summary a number of times, produce a good "rough draft" for review, and even complete a full report with less effort than before. This sense of accomplishment and control led to a proliferation of material. Proposals for new activities, funding grants and applications, publications, research reports, and other documents were initiated by a larger numbers of staff persons, rather than by a few specialists. Workers who had never attempted to publish began to write. Documents, written by hand years before, were "text read" into computer files and easily revamped.

The use of micro-based spreadsheets and databases led professionals to store lists of other professionals and resources in easily recoverable electronic files. Many routine tasks were automated to ease workloads. For example, sample form letters were created and stored where they could be easily modified. A dozen individualized letters could be issued in a few minutes. Composing the newsletter, always a dreaded task, become easier, while its quality improved. In addition, handouts for clients were easily drafted and printed.

The addition of modems allowed professionals to use the telephone to connect to the mainframe and outside bulletin boards, a development which made available new sources of information. National and local bulletin boards included information that was helpful to individuals and clients. Moreover, several practitioners began to use micros to empower their clients. This group experimented by teaching clients to search for information, to learn computer skills, and to survive computer interactions.

Bulletin boards provided the staff with new ideas, from both within and outside their professions. This sort of networking produced novel information exchanges, which led others to perceive the agency as being a valuable source of expertise. Interaction around shared information bases also brought together agencies who had not previously cooperated with one another.

The late adopters remained steadfast in their preference for mainframe computing. Nevertheless, the modems, national databases, and information systems caught their interests. They now had a method for reaching the mainframe via the modem. These individuals began to use the microcomputer as a terminal for the mainframe, in order to do research, data analyses, budgeting, and document preparation. With familiarity, some began to experiment with micros and were soon astonished by the capacity of the little machines. Although the anti-technology group remained, denying the usefulness of computers became harder, and, in the end, those persons had few allies.

CONCLUSION

Computerization of the Midwest Agency occurred in a haphazard fashion. Without formally thinking out the implications of this change, microcomputers were bought at the initial request of a few staff. As new machines were added to do administrative functions (and support staff were required to learn and use them), specific forms of discontent surfaced. And, when microcomputer technology became a national obsession, more machines based on administrative edicts and staff preference were added. A long running and lively debate on the virtues and liabilities of technology began. In any case, the experience of the agency shows that computer technology was not a neutral experience for either practitioners or clients.

The debate over microcomputers was centered on two types of persons: those who were opposed to technology because they believed that computers ran counter to the humanistic values indigenous to a human service profession, allowed the centralization of information and power in the hands of computer specialists, and increased surveillance of professional workers. The other group welcomed computers, particularly the personal computer, as a tool for improving practice, strengthening the independence of workers, reducing centralization and the relevance of administrators, and empowering clients.

The history of computer usage lends support to both points of view. The bulk of the literature seems to be based on the personal experiences of those who believe in technology. Moreover, little has been written about the negative consequences of computer use in the service agencies. Lastly, the literature is noticeably absent on the issue of microcomputers as a force for the oppression of workers and clients.

The experience of the Midwest Agency suggests that whether computers are oppressive or liberalizing depends on a number of variables, including whether: (1) individuals are allowed to computerize at their own pace, (2) training occurs through support groups who help newer users, (3) workers control when and how they use computers, (4) workers have time to "play" and reduce their apprehension, (5) computer-based relationships between support staff and professionals are supported, (6) an atmosphere of information exchange is fostered by administrators, (7) the participation of all levels is sought in the purchase decisions, (8) the recognition exists that no "one best way" exists to initiate computerization, (9) apprehension around new technology is perceived as natural and debate is encouraged, (10) the agency believes that the overeager acceptance of technology is wrong, and (11) the agency realistically portrays the ability of computers and the difficulty in learning to use these machines.

Many of these factors occurred quite by accident in the Midwest Agency. The unplanned evolution of computerization, the dependence on micro technology, and the fiscal limits that made acquisition slow, inadvertently produced many of the key elements that kept computer technology from overwhelming the staff. In addition, the administration's support and openness went a long way in facilitating acceptance by the staff. The tolerant attitude toward resistant groups also helped.

Even though the literature suggests that a rational and planned approach is critical to an organization's success with technology, the Midwest Agency's experience is helpful. Although rational planning should not be abandoned, this strategy must be tempered with the recognition that microcomputers are an innovation. Further, they are a powerful force in the workplace, and thus evoke strong pro and con reactions. The experience with the Midwest Agency leads to the conclusion that any strategy used to introduce computers must take into account the multiple reactions of the staff, the needs of different groups, the recognition that personal computers will and should be individual tools, and the realization that all individuals will approach microcomputers in different ways, at different speeds, and with different results. Microcomputers are a technological innovation, which require that each user be treated as an individual, even those who will never accept this technology.

REFERENCES

Johnson, G. (1986). *Machinery of the Mind.* Redmond WA: Microsoft Press.

9

Human Services and Computers:

Management and Staff Adjustments

Larry Kreuger, MSW, PhD
Assistant Professor of Social Work, University of Missouri

John J. Stretch,, MSW, PhD
Professor of Social Work, Director, Doctoral Program in Social Work, Saint Louis University

INTRODUCTION

The extensive proliferation of computers in the human service field has increased the ability of social work administrators to accomplish their managerial objectives by making large amount of information available in short periods of time. Using this technology for management purposes clearly carries costs and benefits. The shear complexity of computer technology, coupled basic uncertainties common to human service environments, may well lead to organizational decision making based upon less than adequate rationality (Weiner, 1982).

After summarizing the costs and benefits associated with computerized management systems, the authors provide a scheme for analyzing the use of computers by managers and modes of staff adjustment to complex computer technology. These management and staff adjustment strategies arise from the consequences of computerized management systems, as tensions arise over computer access and use. Varying levels of computer expertise among managers and staff sometimes leads to conflict, due to the development of dependency relationships. Each coping strategy varies along four dimensions, involving knowledge of computer hardware, targeted utilization, delegation of authority, and degree of dependence on others. The authors discuss conflicts common to both managers and staff, and offer guidelines for conflict resolution.

COSTS OF AUTOMATED TECHNOLOGY

Initial acquisition costs in time, effort, and resources require decisions for human services managers in the following areas:

1) planning for short and long term agency needs; 2)negotiating acquisition in the turbulent field of rapidly changing computer markets; 3) managing hardware and software compatibility requirements; 4) making decision regarding direct purchase or leasing; 5) security and insurance; 6) access and confidentiality; and 7) renovations required to accommodate computers and staff (Schoech, 1979; Kanter, 1983; Fleischer and Morell, 1985).

In addition to initial acquisition costs, the successful operation of computer technology whether in the form of stand alone or network microcomputers, minicomputers, or mainframe applications, requires further expenditures and extended amounts of organizational effort. Normal wear-and-tear on equipment, software and hardware updates, and specialized supplies require budget increases (Noah, 1978).

In addition to these acquisitions costs, there are continuing organizational costs. These relate to staff training, time required away from routine office activities, down time from equipment failure, regular maintenance, time to backup data, time retrieving lost data, and time spent on routine error checking. All require the attention of human services managers and administrators to keep a computer system's output relevant (Taylor 1981; Krueger, 1987).

Benefits of Automated Technology

The reduction of large amounts of diverse date into meaningful information is the single most important benefit of computer technology (Stretch, 1987). Instantaneous access to data about agency programs, outcomes, and costs associated with service delivery provides administrators with the capability to attend to diverse sets of information with minimal expenditure of energy and time. There is a large variation in the types of answers that can be generated from computerized data bases. Frequency counts, percentages, summary reports, a variety of statistical analyses, and graphics can provide human service managers with a rational understanding of how resources are used and program impact. Additionally, "what if" analyses, using spreadsheet and forecasting software, offer managers a view of potential trouble spots in the future operation of a program (Mental Health Service Systems Reports, 1983).

Computer technology can provide for efficient budgeting, as well as on line analysis of inputs and outputs. Word processing reduces time for the production of printed materials, which tying computers together via networking allows for creation of common data pools. Linkages to outside agencies by modems provides access to other geographic locations. Additionally, linkages to national data bases, user groups and computerized bulletin boards enhance access to outside information sources, and provides managers the opportunity to share data. Pert and Gantt charts track project outcomes and allow for deadlines to be met through managerially controlled monitoring processes (Bresnick, 1983).

The benefits of these technologies involve increased productivity in the performance of routine management tasks. They are also adaptable to specialized tasks in such areas as fund raising, grant writing, and research. Office automation leads to a variety of coping or adjustment practices that are adopted by both management and staff. The authors contend that these strategies develop from the many options available to human service administrators and staff who manage their information through automated technology.

Managerial Modes of Adjustment to Computer Technology

The technology related to data-based, automated office management has grown exponentially in the last ten years. Improvements in micro-processing will continue in the foreseeable future. Growth, however, carries an increased burden for the modern human service administrator (Austin, 1981). Administrators must now decide how much time and energy should be devoted to learning and mastering the plethora of factors associated with modern office automation. A rational coping strategy to increase the limited time available for managers to meet these challenges has arisen from the experience of the authors, as a result of installing management systems in various human services.

There are four basic types of coping adjustments available to a human service manager, in order to keep a modern automated management system operating.

(a) automation expert The automation expert has mastered information technology and routinely uses automated technology in the pursuit of managerial objectives. These managers are conversant with multiple application, costs and benefit trade offs, and user sensitive applications of computer equipment and software. They stay abreast of ongoing computer developments. They review appropriate literature in specialized publications and are knowledgeable about options regarding expandability and compatibility. They benefit from their participation with other computer-oriented managers. Characteristically, they often have personal computers and related equipment at home, and may well be the most knowledgeable computers users in their agency. They can be found as active participants in the Computer Users in Social Services (CUSS) network.

(b) mid level adjuster Characteristically there are managers who have made a concerted effort to master different applications of computer hardware and software. They have stayed conversant with management issues surrounding automation

capabilities. They routinely use one or two software programs for office tasks. These individuals are responsive to new developments in the field. They discuss comfortably the finer points of computing with knowledgeable others. Managers in this category are able to make a wide-range of management decisions with minimal dependence on outside experts.

(c) novice A novice human service computer manager has been introduced to computer equipment, and evidences beginning competence in one or two of the more user friendly programs. The novice manager is also familiar with basic terminology and applications. This manager is greatly dependent upon other computer experts, in order to manage successfully data. Thus the novice manager tends to delegate a great deal of responsibility for routine administration involving computer applications.

(d) uninitiated The uninitiated computer manager has little or no knowledge of computer applications, does not use available technology for performing routine tasks, and is not motivated to spend time and energy learning computer techniques on a first hand basis. This type of manager delegates virtually all responsibility for computers, and is thus almost entirely dependent upon other computer experts.

Table 1 depicts these four types of managers and their respective styles for coping with computer technology.

The managerial challenge illustrated in this model is that adjustments carry varying commitments of time and energy. Each mode of adjustment requires different managerial strategies for dealing not only with routine computer matters but, also, depending upon time commitments, related organizational concerns.

Table 2 summarizes basic managerial approaches in support of coping adjustments.

Additionally, each of the four managerial coping adjustments has consequences with respect to choosing strategies for staff development and staff training.

Table 1. Types of Managerial Coping with Computer Technology

Types of Adjustment	Dimensions of Coping with Automation Technology	
	Knowledge of Equipment Applications	Personal or Business Use
(a) Automation Expert	Extensive	Often
(b) Mid Level Adjust	Moderate	Occasional
(c) Novice	Little	Little
(d) Uninitiated	None	None

Table 2. Managerial Strategies Derived from Coping Adjustments

Types of Adjustment Among Management	Dimensions of Managerial Strategy	
	Dependence on Others	Delegation of Decision Making
(a) Automation Expert	None	Rarely
(b) Mid Level Adjust	Minimal	Split
(c) Novice	Often	Often
(d) Uninitiated	Complete	Total

Staff Modes of Adjustment to Computer Technology

Line and staff workers, like managers, must learn to adjust their work schedules and their time commitments to the requirements of computer technology. Line and staff worker adjustments are similar to those of top management, but tend to be realized along a different set of sub-dimensions:

(a) Power User Adjustment This type of coping is exemplified in computer users who readily absorb new technology and find the learning curve of most software programs to be manageable. These individuals master a wide variety software programs with no difficulty, and readily integrate computer applications into their knowledge base. Typically they want to computerize most routine tasks. These persons run the risk of seeming to overdue both their personal commitment to and personal involvement in these decisions. They may be stereotyped by fellow professionals, because of what their colleagues perceive to be the constant use of jargon. However, these individuals are seen by colleagues as a reliable source of information by those who are having difficulty coping with the demands made by computers. Because of their high level of interest and expertise, power users require no training.

(b) Moderated Adjustment This type of adjustment is manifest in staff and line professionals who have learned one or two software programs. They can handle simple equipment requirements, which allow them to perform straightforward setup tasks and to produce useful but limited output. Moderated adjusters are sufficiently versed in technical language, and thus can communicate fairly well their computer needs to others who have more expertise. These individuals require a moderate amount of training.

(c) Ambivalent Adjustment Like their management counterpart, the ambivalent staff and line adjusters are characterized by a minor interest in computing. They exhibit little practical knowledge of computer hardware and software, and tend to

become marginally involved in one or two computer applications. Ambivalent adjusters require guidance and support from others. They rarely read software documentation manuals. And when they undertake to apply computers to new problems ambivalent users can become an annoyance to other programmers who are more advanced. These ambivalent adjusters thus require maximum training to become minimally functional.

(d) Alienated Adjustment Alienated adjusters are a special category of professionals, who have absolutely no interest in computers. They have no desire to learn basic software programs, and are often threatened by the presence of computer technology in their environment. Those who are alienated find computer applications to be a source of irritation and take pleasure when computer systems breakdown. They require either massive training and a large infusion of managerial support or, from a different management perspective, they may be ignored altogether.

Table 3 provides an overview of the four types of typical staff and line coping adjustments to office automation.

The final component of the proposed analytic scheme involves the interactions among managerial coping adjustments and line-staff coping adjustments. Table 4 summarizes the interaction of management with staff coping adjustments and suggests potential organizational benefits to be derived from the various approaches.

These interactional modes can also be viewed in terms of their potential to engender management and staff conflicts. Conflicts may arise at the personal level at both extremes of the interaction. Managers with high power users. The conflict obtains when management experts become too involved in operations under the control of high power users. A proper balance between the functions of management and the responsibilities of staff would ease, if not eliminate, this sort of conflict. To a lesser degree, the same type of conflict could arise at the other interactional levels in the table.

Conflict is also realized when uninitiated administrators have to manage computer technology with respect to staff who are alienated. Here the conflict cannot be

Table 3. Staff Reactions to Office Automation

Types of Adjustment Among Staff	Dimensions of Coping		
	Extent of Use	Willingness Factor	Training Effort Required
Power User	Extensive	Very Positive	None
Occasional User	Occasional	Positive	Moderate
Ambivalent	Rarely	Mixed	Great deal
Alienated	None	Negative	Mixed*

*Either of two extremes ranging from extensive training and support to complete isolation and thus no training.

Table 4. Organizations Benefits Expected from the Interaction of Management and Staff Coping Adjustments

Staff Coping Adjustments	Managerial Coping Adjustments			
	Automation Expert	Mid Level	Novice	Uninitiated
(potential for organizational benefits)				
Power User	High	High	Moderate	Low
Occasional User	Moderate	Moderate	Low	Very low
Ambivalent	Low	Low	Low	Very low
Alienated	Low	Low	Low	Very low

remedied just by sound management and information clarification. The problems arising from this mode of interaction must be dealt with substantively by providing training and incentives to bring both managers and line-staff personnel to a level of computer sophistication that allows each to perform minimally their respective organizational functions. In both extremes, top management may have to provide direction and solutions for the sake of organizational effectiveness.

Additional management problems that arise include unrealistic expectations for what computers can do, the mystification of both the technology and its application, a reliance on algorithmic decision making, and, in general, an over-reliance on suboptimization at the expense of a systems thinking.

In addition, both managers and staff workers occasionally view computers to have the ability to provide the linkage between answers and questions that is not designed in a data base. This misconception derives from the notion that a computer has the ability to generate original solutions to issues not fully conceptualized. Such an over-determined view can also lead to a reliance on information that already exist in a functioning data base. Such a position is understandable, since it is very difficult to design clean and operationally relevant data bases. Once a data base is constructed, the attendant information is not often examined and, furthermore, is used regularly for purposes unrelated to the design of the original system. This leads to a shortsightedness and an inability to foresee changes in the marketplace, which may in turn impact upon either service delivery or the service appropriateness of an agency (Lauffer, 1984).

Managers are often reluctant to make the investment in initial and continued staff training, and fail to re-invest in both hardware and software components for their computer systems. In order for agencies to receive the considerable benefit associated with computerization, managers must bear the cost of technological and personnel updates. They must also recognize that all hardware and software programs, as well as the personnel who use them, have built in limitations.

In addition to these costs, managers must be prepared to use consultants wisely. Consultants provide objectivity and stimulation for change. Change is inevitable in technology. Thus if human service managers wish to reap the benefits of computers they must be prepared to incur the costs. These costs, however, should be viewed managerially as investment rather than consumption decisions.

Conclusions and Recommendations

The authors have outlined a scheme for analyzing management and staff modes of adjustment to computer technology. The authors contend that managers must seek organizational benefits from the interaction of these modes of adjustment, as a result of sorting through the issues surrounding the level of expertise of both managers and staff personnel and by responding positively to the dependency relationships that may develop. It is characteristic of sound management that resources be managed so that objectives are met. In the final analysis, both managers and line workers must come to view computers as assisting them to best achieve their respective objectives. The following recommendations for managers, from the authors' experience, may provide partial solutions to conflicts arising from the interaction of management and staff coping adjustments:

Options for Managers:

1) Attend local courses (at high school, vocational schools, or colleges and universities) on office automation and computer application;
2) Provide staff with time for both initial and continued computer training;
3) Attend local meetings of a computer user's group to learn of what is going on locally;
4) Include staff members in discussions about office automation and get their recommendations on hardware and software;
5) Subscribe to popular computer journals;
6) Attend introductory courses offered by local vendors to introduce potential purchasers to what equipment can and cannot do;
7) Carefully plan for staff commitments to computer technology;
8) Hire a competent assistant knowledgeable in computer applications:
9) Acquire the services of computer/management consultants.

REFERENCES

Austin, M.J. (1981). *Supervisory Management for the Human Services.* Englewood Cliff,

Bertcher, H.J. (1988). *Staff development in human service organizations.* Englewood Cliff, NJ. Prentice Hall.

Bolter, J.D. (1984). *Turing's man: Western culture in the computer age.* Chapel Hill: The University of North Carolina Press.

Bresnick, D.A. (1983). *Managing the human services in hard times.* New York: NY: Human Services Press.

Calhoun, C.J. (1981). The microcomputer revolution: Technical possibilities and social choices. *Sociological Methods and Research*, 397-437.

Collins, T.W. (1981). Social Science research and the microcomputer. *Sociological Methods and Research* 9 438-60.

Danziger, J.N. (1985). Social science and the social impacts of computer technology. *Social Science Quarterly* 66, Number 1, 3-21.

Fleischer, M. and Morell, J.A. (1985). The organizational and managerial consequences of computer technology. *Computers in Human Behavior* 1 Number 1, 83-93.

Kanter, R.M. (1983). *The change masters.* Beverly Hills, CA: Sage Publications.

Kreuger, Larry and Roy Ruckdeschel (1985). Microcomputers in Human Services Settings: Research Applications. *Social Work* 30, 1, May 1985.

Kreuger, Larry (1987). Microcomputers in Private Practice. *Journal of Independent Social Work* 1 (2), Winter 1987.

Kreuger, Larry and Howard J. Karger. Computers in the 'Not so Human' Services, *Computers in Human Services*, Forthcoming.

Kauffer, A. (1984). *Strategic marketing for not-for-profit organizations: program and resource development.* New York, NY: Free Press.

Lewis, J.A. and M.D. Lewis. (1983). *Management of human service programs.* Monterey, CA: Brooks/Cole Publishing Company.

Mental Health Service System Reports: accounting and budgeting systems for mental health organizations. (1983). Department of Health and Human Services, Rockville, MD.

Morrisey, G.L. (1976). *Management by objectives and results in the public sector.* Reading, MA: Addision Wesley.

Neugeboren, B. (1985). *Organization, policy and practice in the human services.* New York: NY. Longman, Inc.

Noah, J.C. (1978). Information systems in human services: Misconceptions, deceptions, and ethics. *Administration in Mental Health*, 5 Number 2, 99 - 111.

Patti, R.J. (1983). *Social welfare administrations: Managing social programs in a development context.* Englewood Cliffs, NJ. Prentice Hall.

Perrolle, J.A. (1987). *Computers and social change: Information, property, and powers.* Belmont, CA: Wadsworth Publishing Company.

Schoech, D. (1979). A microcomputer based human service information system. *Administration in Social Work* 34 Number 4, 423 - 439.

Stretch, J.J. WIlliam Walker, and M. Unger. (1987). Enhancing ceo's decision making through information systems. *Health Progress* October, 54.

Taylor, J.B. (1981). *Using microcomputers in social agencies.* Beverly Hills, CA: Sage Publications.

Turkle, S. (1984). *The second self: Computers and the human spirit.* New York: Simon and Schuster.

Weiner, M.E. (1982). *Human services management: Analysis and applications.* Homewood, IL: Dorsey Press.

10
Managing Consent in the Computer Age

Terry Holbrook, Ph.D.
Director of Social Work, Willard Psychiatric Center

Not long ago, I read a newspaper story about a social worker, employed by the Welfare Fraud Division of a local Department of Social Services. According to the article, while the worker was on his lunch hour, he saw an attractive young woman, driving a Mercedes. He took down her license number, went back to his office, and using his desk top computer called up on his screen the young woman's vital statistics from the Department of Motor Vehicles. With her social security number, address, birthdate, and a phoney case record number, he was able to find out from various data banks at his disposal (he had to wait one full day for data from the I.R.S.) the woman's marital status, alimony, property, interest income, number of dependents, and, among other things, the fact she had a learning disabled son. He later contacted the woman, posing as an expert on the learning disabled.

While no computer data bank system can ever be made completely fail-safe, or prevent the possible misuse of computerized information by the unethical, there are many technical, administrative, and educative steps that can be taken by social workers in their respective agencies and by schools of social work to help insure confidentiality of client information stored within computerized management information systems (MIS).

Beginning with the Hippocratic Oath, helping professions have agreed that all personal, private information shared or learned about individuals in the course of treatment should be kept strictly confidential (Hunter and Grinnell, 1983). Professions have developed codes of ethics protecting confidentiality, while legal statutes have made the unauthorized disclosure of client information a civil and criminal offense (Reynolds, 1976). Confidentiality is especially crucial for the provision of mental health services, because of the stigma, fear, and social approbrium attached to mental illnesses. It is therefore imperative that social workers begin to educate themselves about the impact of computerization on confidentiality, before an M.I.S. becomes operational.

This chapter will examine one recent, innovative, and comprehensive attempt to develop a computerized tracking system for mental patients in a large urban community in upstate New York. The five year Demonstration Project officially began in 1988, is known as the Integrated Mental Health System (I.M.H.) and is being developed in Rochester, New York, as part of a unique state and local cooperative response to the problems of fragmented mental health service and inadequate funding of community programs for the mentally ill.

INTEGRATED MENTAL HEALTH SERVICES

Discussions of a cooperative effort between state and local government officials and health administrators, in the treatment of the mentally ill in the City of Rochester and Monroe County, began as early as 1959, but had to await passage of the Community Mental Retardation and Mental Health Center Act by Congress in 1963 before funds were actually available. Since that time Rochester has seen the establishment of five community mental health centers, surrounding an urbanly located State inpatient facility. The County Mental Health Board oversees the provision of mental health, mental retardation, alcoholism and substance abuse services in the city and county, and was influential in gaining the cooperation of local officials, the State Legislature, the United Way, and other publically funded service providers in the creation of a single service system. There are presently 16 participating agencies, including community mental health centers, group homes, private mental health clinics, youth services, drug and alcohol treatment and rehabilitation centers, etc., with more expected to join. The Demonstration Project was to develop a computerized tracking system of mental patients and their service providers, in order to plan creatively for and fund services while avoiding the duplication and inefficiencies of the existing uncoordinated delivery system.

Another factor, unique to the Monroe County area that assisted in gaining approval for the Project, was the creation in 1960 of the Monroe County Cumulative Patient Register at the University of Rochester. This was one of the nation's first attempts to collect demographic and diagnostic information on mental patients in an urban area, and provide a pre-existing knowledge base as well as technical expertise in computer technology for the Project. Consequently, the University of Rochester's computers and computer programmers have been largely responsible for the development and implementation of this computerized tracking system (Romano, 1980).

Predictably, given the number of players and the nature of politics, power, and money, many obstacles had to be overcome. While the idea for I.M.H. was conceived in 1979, another seven long years were required for it to gain political and operational support. However, this long delay also allowed for much detailed discussion and planning regarding every aspect of the Project, including debates over the confidentiality of computerized patient information. Subsequently, explicit policy statements, computerized security systems, and detailed procedures were developed to cover all aspects of patient confidentiality. But, before taking a closer look at those policies, procedures, and technical safeguards to confidentiality, the basic M.I.S. software system components developed for I.M.H. must be understood.

First, there is the general System Data File. This is a patient-based file, which contains demographics, client history, service units, cost and revenue information, and evidence of patient participation in all mental health programs.

Second, there is a C.P.S., or Capitation Payment System File, kept on all patients who meet the criteria for inclusion in a unique funding program, designed to overcome major problems resulting from the deinstitutionalization of the chronically mentally ill. By proving an annual sum of money for each patient in the form of a performance contract with the service provider, similar to an H.M.O. (Health Maintenance Organization), prepayment and the increased predictability of funds should allow community providers to plan pro-actively for patients in the community and thereby prevent rehospitalization. Anyway, this is the plan. As will be explained later, this program presented the system with a tough challenge with respect to maintaining client confidentiality.

Finally, there is the Fiscal Data File, a comprehensive journal of fiscal transactions used to manage internal I.M.H. transactions, used to keep track of agency budgets and expenditures. Each participating agency was offered a software package that standardized all these data elements. Information flow into the system included input from the participating agencies based on the System Data File, along with information transfer from the system file in the form of a monthly update to the participating agency. Recognized was that all confidential information remains the property of the patient and the agency.

While the I.M.H. Board is ultimately responsible for screening and approving all requests for analyses, the I.M.H. Data Analysis Committee reviews and approves the day to day information processing. I.M.H. policy states: "to protect data file integrity, individuals or agencies other than I.M.H. data system" (I.M.H. Information Policy and Procedure Manual, 1986: 21). The committee is comprised of representatives from the participating agencies and I.M.H. staff. The committee decides the appropriateness and the priority of information requests, using a four level system for file security level number corresponding to the sensitivity of the information, the committee maintains strict control over what information is released and for what purpose. Level I elements, for instance, pertain to patient identifying information, and are not released under any circumstances.

POLICY: No information sufficient to identify individual patients will be released from the System Data File at any time. Name files required for patient matching will be kept under tight security separate from all other patient and service data, and will not be released for any purpose (I.M.H. Policy Manual, 1986: 23).

All patients' names are scrambled and kept in a separate computer, to which only I.M.H. programmers. As an added precaution, the System Data File is updated in two phases.

> *Phase I* - Each I.M.H. member agency submits information each month regarding patients newly admitted to their facility in the previous month. This file contains identifying information which is used to match new patients to the existing patient name file to determine whether the patient is new to the system. If the patient is new to the system, s/he is assigned a new number. If the patient has already been treated by an I.M.H. agency, the existing ID number is assigned. This number is reinserted into the agency data system, and will be the key to all further processing regarding the patient. Using this approach, the patient identifying information is not stored in conjunction with service or other data, except in the agency system. A facility treating a patient will not know whether that patient is in treatment in another facility unless the patient or other individual tells them (I.M.H. Policy Manual, 1986:23).

This lag time between the submission of data for newly admitted patients and the actual processing of the data by I.M.H. at the end of each month, discourages curious keyboard operators or idle office gossipers from pryng into a client's file, for the only information available at the time of admission is the patient ID number. Phase II is simply the retrieval of patient and service data from agency file tapes. Because there is no interlinking data bank between participating agencies, the I.M.H. member agencies are responsible for delivering their computer tapes to I.M.H. headquarters, where each tape is logged at receipt and dispatch, carefully labeled, and locked in a secure area.

Level II information is facility identifying information, and can only be released with Board approval to designated I.M.H. committees, payers, and the agency itself. All special analyses require written permission, with all requests submitted to the I.M.H. Data Analysis Committee for review and approval. The purpose of the analysis must be specified. Agency identity remains masked, but program and agency designations are made available.

Level III elements are classified as "sensitive information", and include items such as patient symptoms, diagnosis, level of functioning, billing information, and revenues. These factors are released only to designated I.M.H. committees, I.M.H. payers, and the agency. Written permission from an agency is required, and no analysis or files will be generated without a written release of information by a patient.

Finally, Level IV data elements relate to information not classified under the other three levels. Again, the Board must also approve the release of these data.

Probably the most difficult confidentiality policy and procedure for I.M.H. to develop involved C.P.S. patients. The reader may recall the Capitation Payment

System (C.P.S.) was designed to assist in tracking chronically mentally ill patients in the community. This entailed the development of individual contracts for care of specified patients by community mental health centers (lead agencies), based on the patient's prior utilization of State inpatient mental health services. Accordingly, a sufficient amount of identification must be kept on file, so that other agencies can determine whether or not a patient should be returned to the lead agency. All C.P.S. patients, therefore, are required to sign a special release form. This document specifies the use of the information, and covers the release of information necessary for C.P.S. care. Patients unwilling to sign such a release will not be enrolled. The data file on C.P.S. patients is accessible only to participating I.M.H. agencies. Regular reports of C.P.S. patients activities are for I.M.H. and lead agency use only. Individual summaries will not be released unless the contracted lead agency has obtained patient consent in advance, in writing. A separate release form will be obtained for any C.P.S. evaluation or research study.

To date, no one has actually been enrolled in the C.P.S. program, and thus is difficult to say how these special precautions will be managed by social workers, whose job it is to cajole, convince, and persuade patients to sign on the dotted line. Of the approximately 20,000 people receiving mental health services in Monroe County each year, only 300 are eligible for the C.P.S. program. Still, the benefits to chronic patients from an integrated single service system, modeled on the Health Maintenance Organization concept, seems to outweigh the risks. As the previous discussion illustrates, computer technology can be made relatively safe for human consumption, provided enough attention is given to confidentiality procedures and security. What remains problematic, however, is the human element.

TEACHING COMPUTER ETHICS

Just as no one person can plan for every conceivable contingency, preventing unethical social workers, or other dubiously motivated persons, from misusing computerized information is difficult. However, schools of social work could do better in recognizing and teaching students and practitioners about the ethical concerns related to confidentiality and computerized information. While there will always be an occasional worker who abuses his or her professional trust, there are probably many more who simply do not appreciate the power of the computer and their relationship to this technology. As many social critics of technological change have observed (Stanley 1978, Winner 1977), machines do our bidding. It is people who decide these devices will be used and for what purpose. Consequently, practitioners have an ethical responsibility to understand and inform their clients about how confidential information is protected by computers, as well as the threats to privacy. Simply because computers are machines that lack the capacity for individualized judgment and reason, does not mean that manual record keeping systems offer better protection of confidential information.

Anyone who has worked in a social agency, hospital, or business, is aware of the daily breaches in confidentiality with manual filing systems. A chart delivered to the wrong place, progress notes misfiled, insurance forms copied and lost or sent to the wrong address, or a chart misplaced or left on someone's desk are daily occurrences. With the vast increase in persons seeking information, including regulatory agencies, peer review teams, auditors, third party payers, researchers, representatives of courts, clinicians, and clerical staff, the computer offers the best way to limit the number of hands a chart must pass through in a given day. Increased control is provided over those who have access to information along with greater accuracy improved filing capacity. Whereas computers require sign on and off codes, security clearances, pass words, and the like, existing manual systems usually require a single signature on a routine request. Even though computers offer "instantaneous access" to confidential information to those possessing the knowledge to enter the system, there is a lot to know and thus a greater chance of being caught without proper authorization or education. Still, the perceived threat that computers pose to personal privacy has generated many of the arguments against the computerization of records.

The real argument, however, is not with the technology, but with the attitudes, training, and understanding of those service providers and organizations who are assigned to collect and protect information. Because of the efficiency of computers in processing and storing personal information, the attitudes and safeguards associated with manual filing systems are inappropriate for this technology.

The members of the I.M.H. Project recognized this increased responsibility and planned accordingly. The social work profession also needs to plan for computerized record keeping systems and to begin raising the level of consciousness of practitioners regarding confidentiality and the computer.

MANAGING "INFORMED CONSENT"

Perhaps because of fears of "Big Brother", computer phobia and a growing recognition of the importance of records in modern society, Congress began examining recently the need for legislation that protects individual privacy. In 1967, Congress held a series of subcommittee hearings on the growing use of computers and their perceived threat to privacy, as guaranteed in the Constitution (U.C.L.A. Law Review, 1968).

As a result of these hearings and others held by the Privacy Protection Study Commission, Federal legislation was passed in 1974 that all federally funded programs had to abide by these privacy rules and regulations or risk losing Federal funding. The Act was designed to protect consumers of all government funded services from having their records released without their knowledge. A written release was now required that specified the agency to whom information was to be released, the purpose, and the type of data, as well as a time limit for authorization, moreover, this release could be withdrawn by a client at any time. In many States, including New York, this Federal legislation was followed by Personal Privacy and Protection Laws, which extended this protection even further. For example, patients for the first time could have access to their own medical records.

Although written releases of confidential information had been required for years at many social agencies, clients now have legal recourse to see and to amend their records, if necessary. The fact remains, however, that very few consumers ever ask to see their records and continue to sign releases of information to unspecified others. This is because clients believe signing these forms is required for them to receive services, and are generally ignorant of these new legal protections. According to one of the leading experts on confidentiality in social work: "most settings realize the need to obtain written consent for release of information. However, many social work settings and those of other disciplines as well, have handled this process in such a way that its very purpose is effectively sabotaged" (Wilson, 1978:58). The author goes on to describe the use of "blanket forms", incompletely filled out by the worker, with signed extra copies so the client will not have to complete another document. In the age of the computer, workers must be retrained and remotivated to treat the issue of "consent" with the respect and attention it deserves. Social work ethics courses should be using case studies of computer confidentiality violation, in order to alert workers to the increased legal and ethical responsibility assumed when they present a client with a release form for computerized records.

As the I.M.H. Project illustrates, written releases of information are crucial to the integrity of the system. If patients sign a release to participate in a program, or agree to share their personal history, number of hospital admissions, symptoms, diagnosis or whatever else with a legitimate service provider, they have a legal right to know the conditions under which this information may be released to researchers or other parties. If written releases are not sufficiently explained or are treated as merely routine, the social workers who represent agencies or computerized tracking systems could find themselves explaining to an angry client or unsympathetic lawyer their lack of regard for confidential information. Historically, the courts have been very careful to protect individual privacy rights, despite the well meaning intentions of service providers (Wilson, 1978:60). Moreover, not only individual practitioners must understand the importance of confidentiality in the age of the computer, social service and mental health organizations must also recognize this issue.

CONFIDENTIALITY AND BUREAUCRACY

According to Michael Lipsky (1980:57):

> Most encounters with bureaucracy appear to be characterized by consent, but the structure of choices available to the clients limits the range of alternative behaviors that they consider realistically available. In short, client consent is continuously being managed by public agencies.

In most human service agencies, social workers are assigned the task of effectively managing client consent. The use of blanket consent forms, treating the consent form as a requirement rather than a choice, minimizing the quantity or kinds of information to be released, and including the consent forms among other routine papers for signature, are all familiar techniques for managing client consent. Social workers may feel that in order for services to be adequately rendered, obtaining information from other agencies is necessary, justified, and in the client's best interest.

Often social workers are faced with clients who would rather starve than accept welfare, freeze to death rather than live in a shelter, or commit suicide rather than agree to mental health services. Social workers are confronted daily with ethical decisions that have immediate, far reaching, and serious implications for clients' lives. Protecting patient confidentiality, especially from other service providers, may seem like an unnecessary waste of time and counter productive. It is easier to treat confidentiality protection as a minor inconvenience, thereby requiring routine signatures rather than taking the time to explain in detail each request for information and the risks of refusal. After all, human service agencies would not be able to function without client consent. Programs would be disrupted, budgets challenged, and research stymied if clients refused to release confidential information. Perhaps this is why many human service agencies have given their tacit approval to sloppy client consent management practices. Generally, small breaches in confidentiality procedures work in favor of the client, and only the rare exception gets publicity or court attention. Like so many other facts of modern life, records and the need for records has become taken for granted. Therefore, concern for the concomitant need for confidentiality is overlooked, unless there is a legal problem or a serious breach of confidentiality. While the increased danger of automated records and breaches of confidentiality have been recognized, these dangers are not viewed as stemming from the lax practices and attitudes toward the confidentiality of manual record keeping systems. In 1973, N.A.S.W. created guidelines for the use of automated record keeping systems. These recommendations included prohibiting the use of secret records, restricting the use of universal identifiers such as social security numbers, and sharing information without the consent of clients. However, as Wilson noted, the N.A.S.W. policy failed to specifically recognize the client's right to grant permission for data to be stored in the first place (Wilson, 1978:47). Social workers seem to be trying to solve the confidentiality questions of the future in terms of the practices accepted in the past. This could prove exceedingly problematic, as clients become more aware of their rights surrounding the issue on confidentiality.

In one recent study of the requests for release of the records of psychiatric patients, although most patients felt strongly about limiting access to records, 81% felt that release was mandatory. The majority also believed only doctors and nurses could see their records, and only 16% knew of any legal requirements to safeguard confidentiality. The authors concluded:

> this situation, coupled with the fact that most patients have inadequate knowledge of the content of their records, essentially renders the patient's release of medical records uninformed and involuntary (Kinzie, Holmes and Arent, 1985:843-846).

An earlier study of psychiatric patients' knowledge of confidentiality protections found similar results, with 83% reporting they did not know of any rules or laws regulating who had access to their hospital charts. These same patients, however, felt very strongly that access should be limited to their records, and stated they would be very angry if information was released without their permission. The same study also found that even though patients were surprisingly willing to share private information with other professions, "factors that diminish confidentiality in psychiatric care may impair the willingness of patients to seek and remain in treatment" (Schmid et al, 1983:355). Of course, this is one of the primary justifications the courts have cited for recognizing the privilege of confidential communication.

It would seem that a massive re-education campaign is needed to focus attention on both the existing practices and the belief systems of clients and human service organizations, concerning the confidentiality of record keeping in general and the challenges of confidential computerized records in particular. Unless such re-education is undertaken, computer technology could experience an unnecessary and irrational setback. This reversal may not be due to the technology, but a possible backlash of angry patients upon learning about their legal rights to confidentiality, their misguided faith in manual record keeping systems, and their distrust of computer technology. Of course, some may fear that by focusing attention on the process of consent and informing patients of their legal rights to confidentiality and record access, clients may be unduly alarmed and refuse to sign the required release forms. I feel the greater risk relates to the loss of confidence among clients, who, upon learning of their rights from other sources, will either be misinformed or conclude that their therapists and the State have deliberately deceived them. While clients who are fearful of computer technology may indeed refuse to sign release forms, at least someone will have spent the time to explain both their rights and some of the advantages of computers over manual record keeping systems in protecting confidentiality. Given repeated explanations, in an open, informative, and trusting atmosphere, fearful clients may reconsider their views. To be realistic, the alternative must also be evaluated —clients may refuse to sign consent to release information forms and disrupt the delivery of services.

Client related information is vital to operating a human service organization. Failure to recognize that trust in the confidentiality of case records allows this information to flow, is a fatal flaw that will only be compounded by the introduction of computer technology. The real or perceived loss of control over confidential information stored in computers may result in a much more careful and skeptical public reaction to the present "managed" consent practices of public service bureaucracies. What was easily managed yesterday may not be so easily managed tomorrow, especially when computer technology, with its attendant fears, is added to the confidentiality equation. Unless social workers begin to educate their clients, the public, and their employers to the dangers posed by a loss of confidence in confidentiality safeguards, especially with regard to computer technology, practitioners may find ourselves in a very difficult and defensive situation.

While human service organizations may have other legitimate organizational goals, such as the need to establish eligibility, prevent fraud, improve cost effectiveness, etc., the basic trust of the clients in the confidentiality practices of an agency allows the treatment process to continue. Without this trust, the smooth flow of vital client information for planning and treatment purposes will discontinue, along with funding, programs, and payrolls. Time spent with a client to make sure he/she understands the process related to the release of information is labor intensive and costly. It may also be costly to educate clients about their right to confidentiality and to present a balanced discussion of computerized record protections. However, the cost of not doing so may be greater in the long run. In the words of one advocate of computer records, "money spent for improved security is not available for other uses, such as patient care and data analysis" (Wolkon and Lyon, 1986:11). While record security and confidentiality must compete with other organizational needs and values for fiscal resources, managers and clinicians alike must recognize the importance of confidentiality or everyone loses.

THE STATE v. CONFIDENTIALITY

Ironically, the Federal, State and local government are both the greatest advocates and the greatest potential violators of client confidentiality. The government's need for information pertaining to taxation, public safety, and national security seems almost unsatiable. Some writers have estimated that the government has as many as ten to twenty dossiers on every average American (Wilson, 1978). For those Americans who have had the misfortune of having to apply for welfare, or suffer from a mental illness or some other disability, the number of records increases proportionately to the services sought. Yet these same citizens are the ones who are the least educated about their rights regarding confidentiality, and are most vulnerable to an invasion of their privacy. For example, officials from New York State Office of Mental Health believed that because they were paying for the I.M.H. project, they should have direct access to I.M.H. computers, in order to use the service pattern information to develop cost effectiveness ratios for other communities and plan for the State-wide implementation of similar programs. Also requested were computer printouts for a variety of non-project related information, such as the service utilization rate for criminal procedure law patients (C.P.L.). Fortunately, the State representative had only one vote on the Project Data Advisory Committee and their requests were denied.

The impulse to collect and use computerized information for other than its intended purpose remains strong, especially when the request comes from a powerful funding agency whose stated objective is the improvement of service officials misusing computerized data on private citizens for a host of ostensibly good reasons. This danger, of course, has sparked much of the legislation and negative publicity surrounding computer technology, and requires that practitioners become more sensitive to the possible conflicts of interest that may develop even regarding the authorized utilization of computerized data. The fact remains, social workers have more to lose than they will gain by inadvertently breaching the trust of clients. Moreover, once patient information is accumulated on a computer disk, the risk that existing legal protections might be relaxed must be considered. For example, in 1973 the State of Maine proposed that the Attorney General should have complete access to the records of all public agencies, in order to properly carry out the functions of his office. The purpose of the bill was to avoid the expense to taxpayers of subpoenaing people and papers. Fortunately, the bill was defeated (M.D.L.R., 1977:340). Similar bills in other states have been more successful. New York State, for example, recently amended its confidentiality statutes to allow the Department of Corrections to have access to the Department of Mental Health records without the consent of inmates, ostensibly to provide an appropriately secure facility (Mental Hygiene Law Section 33:13 (C) - 1985). Public safety is always a potent legal argument for breaching the confidentiality of individuals, and thus has had frequent success in State legislatures. Computerized records make those exclusions or exceptions much more efficient, comprehensive, and possibly more devastating. Thus, teachers in Schools of Social Work and practitioners must be aware of the most recent confidentiality legislation, and be able to inform clients about any changes in the law prior to a release of information. Mandatory reporting of child abuse cases or the duty to warn others of threats to harm by those in treatment are well known examples. Since many states do not offer statutory protection for social workers under privileged communication, practitioners should be prepared to alert clients to the relevant confidentiality statutes and requirements. The time and effort involved informing patients of legal protection and mandatory reporting requirements is well worth the possible cost to the client of subpoenaed computerized records.

In New York State, the courts have ruled that identifying the diagnostic information of clients served by a drug rehabilitation agency was not a violation of confidentiality, simply because these data were stored in a computerized system. The legal argument maintained that the agency's objective was treatment not punishment, and the public's right to know how its money was being spent outweighed the individual interest in privacy, unless a specific breach of confidentiality could be proven (Wilson, 1978:44).

Recently, however, that argument has been successfully challenged. A Massachusetts Supreme Court decision (Commonwealth v Kobrin, 1985) ruled that the State did not have the authority to require the complete case record of psychiatric patients for investigating Medicaid fraud. In the past, most notably Camperlengo v. Blum, the courts ruled that the federal statute for the disclosure of complete records for Medicaid investigations preempted the State's law of privilege (Appelbaum, 1986:334). Because the courts are frequently reviewing and re-interpreting what is meant by privilege and confidentiality, social workers must keep abreast of these issues before rather than after an M.I.S. system goes on line (see Mental Disability Law Reporter, 1977, 337-354).

COMPUTER CONFIDENTIALITY AND SOCIAL WORKERS

If for no other reason than self-protection, social workers must be more aware of the need for strict enforcement and compliance with existing confidentiality protections, procedures, and precautions, especially with computerized record keeping systems. Whereas social workers are presently part of the problem, they can also become the targets of confidentiality abuses.

In 1986, Congress passed the Health Care Quality Improvement Act. This new legislation has called for the creation of a national computerized data bank containing a physician master file. This master file would be used by hospital administrators to check the current license, qualifications, and credentials of physicians applying for positions. Additionally, peer review activities and disciplinary proceedings would be included. While the law gives physicians the right to review and amend all the information on file, the physician must rely on the confidentiality procedures, security clearance policies, and the judgment of clearinghouse officials to release the necessary information to the right people. Given the high stakes and possible damage to professional reputations, physicians are understandably concerned about the existence of a national computer system. While the new law tried to allay the concerns of the American Medical Association over proper access to confidential information by imposing a $10,000 dollar fine for violations, physician were not reassured (Iglehart, 1987:960-964).

Since the precedent has been set, soon other health care professions, including social work, will be required to do the same. Will social workers trust their agencies' personnel offices, or be as confident about confidentiality protections as their clients are expected to be? Or will social workers, because of their knowledge and experience with signed releases and informed consent, demand more stricter controls and more detailed policies protecting their own right to privacy?

Because computer technology tends to blur the distinction between public and private information, while appearing and disappearing at the push of a button, social workers need to remind themselves continually of the importance of confidentiality in their daily transactions with clients. Computers offer convenience, efficiency, and control, but unless social workers practice confidentiality and actually seek to influence human service administrators to pay the cost of adequately protecting computerized records, the dangers of manual record keeping systems will only be multiplied by the speed and efficiency of the new technology.

The computer can be programmed to protect confidential information, as well as instantaneously divulge data. This technology can be used to increase the reliability and accuracy of the information that is recorded by cross-checking and referencing. The chances of unauthorized disclosure can also be reduced, through elegant security systems. Ultimately, however, people, not the computer, will decide how much privacy is worth.

BIBLIOGRAPHY

Appelbaum, P. S. (1986). "Confidentiality: Winning for a Change." *Hospital and Community Psychiatry*, Volume 37, 334-335.

"Computerization of Government Files: What Impact on the Individual?" (1968). *U.C.L.A. Law Review* 15, 1371-1498.

Hunter, M. S., and Grinnel, R. N. Jr. (1983). "Social Workers' Perceptions of *Privacy: A Research Note.*" Social Work, v 28, 68-69.

Iglehart, J. K. (1987). "Congress Moves to Bolster Peer Review: The Health Care Quality Improvement Act of 1986." *The New England Journal of Medicine*, v 316, 960-964.

Integrated Mental Health Inc. (1986). "Plan for Confidentiality of Information." Rochester, New York: I.M.H. Confidentiality Plan.

Kinzie, J. D., Holmes, J. L., and Arent, J. (1985) "Patients' Release of Medical Records: Involuntary Uninformed Consent?" *Hospital and Community Psychiatry*, v36, 843-847.

Lipsky, M. (1980). *Street Level Bureaucracy*. New York: Russell Sage Foundation.

Mental Disability Law Reporter. (1977). "Legal Issues in State Mental Health Care: Proposals for Change", (Therapeutic Confidentiality), 337-354.

Reynolds, M. M. (1976). "Threats to Confidentiality." *Social Work*, vol. 21, No. 2, pp. 108 - 113.

Romano, J. (1980). "Twenty-five Years Later." *Psychiatric Quarterly*, v52,7-22.

Stanley, M. *The Technological Conscience*. Chicago: The University of Chicago Press, 1978.

State of New York. Mental Hygiene Law Section 33.13 (C) 9. Amendment to the law governing confidentiality of patient records, effective Sept. 1985. Senate-Assembly Session March 26, 1985.

Wilson, S. J. (1978) *Confidentiality in Social Work*. New York: The Free Press.

Winner, L. (1977). *Autonomous Technology*. Cambridge: The MIT Press.

Wolkon, G. H. and Lyon, M. (1986). "Ethical Issues in Computerized Mental Health Data Systems." *Hospital & Community Psychiatry*, v 37, 11- 16.

11

The Utilization of Computers in Social Service Agencies

John T. Pardeck, MSW, PhD
Professor and Chair, Department of Social Work, Southeast Missouri State University

Karen Collier Umfress
Arkansas State University

John W. Murphy
Associate Professor of Sociology, Miami University

Once thought of as the exclusive property of business and government, computers are now appearing in social service agencies. Currently, the typical use of computers in social service agencies is for information management (Gripton, 1983). This usage is largely for indirect practice activities and normally involves only a small number of administrative personnel.

As computer technology increases in sophistication and becomes less expensive, other aspects of service delivery will be undertaken via the computer. For example, many software programs are now available for conducting the initial interview with clients, and others can be used to perform clinical testing, diagnosis, and even consultation. However, Gripton (1983) points out that only a small number of social service agencies use these newer technologies. Even though a technological *ethos* pervades society and computer hardware and software continue to proliferate, this technology is underutilized. Gripton's discovery has been corroborated by research undertaken in industry, where only elementary operations are regularly computerized. (Majchrzak, Nieva, and Newman, 1986).

Several factors have been cited to explain the limited use of computer technology in direct practice activities. One is that very few articles on computer technology have been published in the social work literature over the last two decades. One study reported that only 31 articles on computer technology were published in the eight leading social work journals from 1970 to 1976 (Boyd, Hylton, & Price, 1978). More recent research by Murphy and Pardeck (1986a, 1986b) found that even in the 1980s very few articles appeared. Thus, the paucity of articles may both reflect and be contributing to the current lack of knowledge among social service personnel about the potential usefulness of computer technology not only for administration and research, but in interviewing and clinical testing.

Another factor may be the limited training available to social work graduate students. Specifically, very few programs require courses in computer technology (Pardeck, 1988). This is due in part to the lack of emphasis placed on the critical evaluation of intervention. Without an appreciation for research, computers will not likely be viewed as having much utility. (Pardeck & Murphy, 1986).

A final factor in the lack of understanding, if not outright resistance to this technology, is the value base of the social work profession. Clearly, the profession is based predominately on humanistic values, which require a client-centered orientation (Federico, 1980). Through the evolution of social work theory and practice, an ideology has emerged which suggests that computers are intrinsically harmful to clients (Gripton, 1983). A number of writers have argued that the resistance to computer technology will not abate in social work until social workers receive a sophisticated introduction to computerization. At present, there is some evidence that social work educational programs are beginning to include courses on computer technology at the graduate level (Pardeck, 1988). If this trend continues, negative attitudes toward computer technology may begin to change.

With regard to this last point, Munson (1988) has noted that courses related to the use of computers can be taught in a variety of ways. Emphasis can be placed on either the logistics or the philosophy of computerization. At this time, the focus appears to be the mastery of technique. And as long as this is the case, insight into how computers can be used in a socially sensitive manner will probably not be acquired.

In view of the underutilization of computer technology, the present research seeks to identify the availability of computer technology in social service agencies and to explore the perceptions of computers by social service personnel, in particular social workers. Perceptions of computers by social workers are assessed in terms of their level of understanding of and attitudes toward this technology. The obvious implication of this research is that if social workers are found to be lacking in appreciation of computer technology, as suggested by the literature, and if they have a negative attitude toward computers, the use of this technology will not necessarily improve the delivery of social services. Funds will be wasted on new equipment and faulty practices.

This study is more extensive than previous ones. In addition to gathering information pertaining to how practitioners understand the possible uses of computers, questions were asked related to training. The attempt was made to gain insight into both theoretical and practical matters.

METHOD

The population surveyed was 490 licensed certified social workers in a mid-southern state in the United States. One hundred of the social workers were randomly selected to serve as the research sample, and a questionnaire was sent to each during the Spring of 1986. A total of 59 social workers returned the questionnaire. The average age of the social workers who responded was 44 years. Over half of the respondents were female. The majority were white. Over 90% of the respondents possessed a Master of Social Work degree (See Table I).

The research questionnaire consisted of 34 items. Ten of the items in Likert-scale form were designed to measure attitudes toward computer technology; each item consisted of a 4-point scale ranging from (1) Strongly Agree to (4) Strongly Disagree. Content validity of the questionnaire was established through a pretest conducted on six randomly selected professional social workers employed in social service agencies. The workers participating in the pretest agreed that the instrument was clearly written and had validity.

RESULTS

As can be seen in Table II, 76% of the social workers surveyed had a computer in their agency; 38% used the computer as part of their practice. Table II suggests many of the agencies that employed social workers used time sharing, since 25% had access to a mainframe computer system. Only 12% of the workers utilized the micro computer. One of the more noteworthy findings is that only 12% of the workers used computer technology on a daily basis, and that 35% never used the computer. One clear implication is that most agencies have computer technology available to workers, but the majority of the workers did not use the technology.

Table III indicates the type of support these practitioners received with regard to preparing them to use a computer. Only 7% of the social workers surveyed had an

Table 1 Demographic Characteristics

Sex		Race	
Female	56 %	Black	9 %
Male	44 %	White	86 %
		Other	5 %
		Professional degree	
Average age	44 Years	MSW	95 %
		Other	5 %

Table II Computer Technology In Agency (Percentages)

Question	Response	%
Computer in Agency	Yes	76
	No	15
	NR	9
Computer Used as Part of your Practice	Yes	38
	No	40
	NR	22
Type of Computer in Agency	Micro	12
	Mainframe	25
	Micro and Mainframe	10
	Other	10
	NR	43
Frequency of Computer Usage	Daily	12
	1 to 4 Times a Week	7
	Monthly	7
	Time Varies	3
	Never	35
	NR	38

NR = No Response

educational experience that prepared them to use computer technology; however, 35% did have in-service training on computer technology. This training ranged from 1-10 hours for 23% of the social workers to more than 10 hours for 17% of them. Interestingly, 64% of the social workers felt that computer technology should be included in professional social work education; 67% reported that in-service training should be available in the agency.

Table IV illustrates a number of important findings pertaining to the ways computer technology is used in the agency. The most common use is for storing and retrieving records; 40% checked this item. Twenty-nine percent implemented computer technology for program evaluation and other types of research. Only 21% used computer technology for letter writing, which is an unexpected finding. Since word processing programs are readily available and are user friendly, one would think that most of the social workers surveyed would be using computer technology for such a routine activity.

It is not surprising to find that only 3% of the workers used the computer for conducting therapy or that 7% utilized it for the in-take interview (see Table IV). As suggested earlier, a number of writers have reported that social workers as a

Table III Training In Computer Technology

Question	Response (%),+					
Did your professional education in social work prepare you to use a computer?	Yes	7	No	86	NR	7
Have you received in-service training on computer usage?	Yes	35	No	60	NR	5
Number of hours of in-service training received	0	60	1–10	23	10+	17
Should training in computer technology be included in professional social work education?	Yes	64	No	17	NR	19
Should training in computer technology be included as part of in-service training?	Yes	67	No	14	NR	19

NR = No Response

professional group have not begun to tap the potential for computer usage in therapy or other micro-level intervention activities (Pardeck & Murphy, 1986). This is clearly illustrated in Table IV.

With regard to attitudes toward computers, some extremely important data were uncovered. Even though social workers have little or no training in computer technology, the responses to Question 1 indicate that 64% either agreed or strongly agreed that computers can improve their effectiveness (see Table V). No doubt, this attitude is heavily influenced by the current evolution toward a high-tech society that often unquestioningly accepts most technological innovations (Ihde, 1982). However, the responses to Question 2 imply that this attitude does not carry over to the use of computers in therapy.

Table IV The Ways Computer Technology Is Used In Agency

Use of computer	%
Letter writing	21
Writing case records	12
Storing and retrieving client records	40
Monitoring a client's treatment plan	19
Planning and organizing the agency's budget	24
Administering and scoring clinical tests	5
Conducting in-take interviews	7
Program evaluation or other types of research	29
A tool for conducting therapy session	3

Table V Attitudes Towards Computers

Question	Replies (%)				
	SA	A	D	SD	NR
1. Do computers improve the effectiveness of social workers?	17	47	17	8	14
2. Can computers actually do therapy?	0	7	21	58	14
3. Does a computer help a social worker to manage information effectively?	38	46	2	2	12
4 Have computers removed the human element from social service delivery?	4	10	38	34	14
5. Are computers a threat to client confidentiality?	10	38	29	7	16
6. Do computers assist practitioners in assessing a client's problems?	5	50	19	8	12
7. Is organizational efficiency increased through the use of computers?	36	41	3	8	12
8. Does the use of computers enable practitioners to assist an increased number of clients?	10	41	29	6	14
9. Will computers drastically change the nature of social work?	9	16	48	12	17
10. The dignity of clients is jeopardized by computers.	5	12	53	14	16

SA = Strongly Agree; A = Agree; D = Disagree; SD = Strongly Disagree; NR = No Response

Another significant attitude uncovered is that the social workers are very concerned about confidentiality (Table V). A number of researchers have reported that psychiatrists and psychologists also have similar concerns about the threat posed by the computer to client confidentiality (Pardeck, 1988). However, the responses to Question 10 suggest that the dignity of clients is not threatened by computers. This appears to be somewhat of a paradox, given the strong feelings about the threat of computers to confidentiality.

The responses to Question 9 imply that the majority of the social workers surveyed did not feel that computers will drastically change the nature of social work. This finding is ironic, given the fact that computers have the potential to dehumanize the work place (Murphy, Pardeck, Nolden, & Pilotta, 1987), and that most of the social workers surveyed had little or no understanding of computer technology and its implications. Even though computer technology can greatly increase the efficiency of the workplace, it is imperative that social workers understand that it must be used responsibly (Pardeck, 1988). Such use occurs only if social workers are thoroughly trained in computer technology, which they clearly are not, and if this training emphasizes the benefits and costs (Murphy & Pardeck, 1986b).

CONCLUSIONS AND IMPLICATIONS

The results of this study for the most part are consistent with other research on computers and social workers. According to the findings: (1) social workers have limited understanding of computer technology; (2) social service agencies have not begun to use computer technology to its fullest potential; (3) social workers have received little training in computer technology through the professional social work curriculum; and (4) social service agencies do not provide in-service training on computer technology.

The attitudes of social workers toward computers were somewhat unexpected. In particular, they had very positive attitudes as to the assets of computer technology. However, strong doubts were noted concerning computer use in therapy, and the questions raised in the area of confidentiality. These doubts appear consistent with the humanistic base of professional social work.

A number of important implications for the professional social worker also were uncovered. There is a need for the curriculum to incorporate courses on computer technology. In addition, agencies should provide social workers with in-service computer training, which would lead to increased understanding of the technology and allow the social worker to develop important skills in its use. However, it is important that the training take into account the tremendous potential of the computer to dehumanize the worker and client relationship.

REFERENCES

Boyd, L., Hylton, J., & Price, S. (1978). Computers in social work practice: A review. *Social Work*, 23, 368-371

Federico, R. *The social welfare institution* (1980). (3rd ed.). Lexington, MA: D. C. Health and Company.

Gripton, J. (1983). Computerizing your practice. *Practice Digest*, 6, 16-20.

Ihde, D. (1982). *Historical-ontological priority of technology over science*. Paper presented at the International Conference of Philosophy and Science in Phenomenological Perspective.

Majchrzak, Anne, Nieva, Veronica, and Newman, Paul (1986). "Adoption and Use of Computerized Manufacturing Technology: A National Survey." In *Managing Technological Innovation*, by Donald D. Davis and Associates (pp.105-126). San Francisco: Jossey-Bass.

Munson, Carlton E. (1988). "Microcomputers in Social Work Education" *Computers and Human Services* 3(1/2), 143-157.

Murphy, J., & Pardeck, J.(1986a). Computerized clinical practice: Promises and shortcomings. *Psychological Reports*, 59, 1099-1113.

Murphy, J., & Pardeck, J. (1986b). Technology and the manufacture of madness: A new dimension. *International Journal of Social Psychiatry*, 32(2), 41-46.

Murphy, J., Pardeck, J., Nolden, W., & Pilotta, J. (1987). Conceptual issues related to the use of computers in social work practice. *Journal of Independent Social Work Practice*, 1(4), 63-73.

Pardeck, J. (1987). Microcomputer technology in clinical practice: An analysis of ethical issues. *Journal of Independent Social Work Practice*. 2, 71-81.

Pardeck, J., & Murphy, J. (1986). Micro computer technology in clinical social work practice: Benefits and problems. ARETE, 11, 35-42.

12

Important Non-Technical Considerations in the Development of an MI System

John W. Murphy, PhD
Associate Professor of Sociology, Miami University

John T. Pardeck, MSW, PhD
Professor and Chair, Department of Social Work, Southeast Missouri State University

At this time program evaluation is viewed to be an important enterprise in most social service programs. Because of this, managers are scrambling to collect numerous types of information that were never before gathered in a systematic manner. Due to this increased demand for information, efficient methods must be sought for collecting, storing, and utilizing the data that are required to evaluate the effectiveness of service delivery. Moreover, improved management decisions are thought to follow from the development of a management information system (MIS). The MIS, therefore, is understood to be necessary for handling the information that is required currently to be an effective manager. Specifically, the belief is that a MIS will enable data to be processed efficiently and in novel ways. While this may be true, special care must be taken to insure that a MIS is properly installed and maintained, or the resulting system will be of little use in operating a program (Murphy, Pardeck, Nolden, and Pilotta, 1987).

At this juncture, the reader needs to be reminded that most often technical issues are the focus of MIS development. Clearly this trend is consistent with the "technological imperative" that underpins modern societies. What is meant by this theme is that through technological control, any task can be replaced by technical operations whenever possible. Data collection, accordingly, is assumed to be more effective and efficient when this process is mechanized. When the use of data is routine, or unaffected by situational contingencies, mistakes are reduced and patient care improves. Yet as Ashley Montagu quipped recently, the use of computers cannot be characterized by the phrase "garbage in, Gospel out" (Murphy and Pardeck, 1988). His point is that technological machinations are no substitute for sound methodological practices and managerial insight. In other words, practitioners should not be so enamored of information technology that they forget an important lesson. That is, technical operations are sustained by human judgments. The human side of installing a MIS must not be overlooked.

A management information system may be simply defined as a systematic, standardized method for collecting, organizing, storing, and utilizing data (Murphy, 1981). In terms of conducting program evaluation, for example, information about patients, service delivery, staff activities, and finances must be readily available. Instead of having this information located in different locations throughout an organization, data are centralized by a MIS and made easily accessible. A MIS, therefore, is typically thought to be the key to improving service delivery. Yet information is always context-bound, or located within a network created by policies, judgments, and concerns. The result of forgetting this simple idea may be that a technically sound MIS will be rendered dysfunctional.

What should be remembered is that there are no shortcuts to developing a properly functioning MIS. No-one should rush into the process of developing such a system without a few rules that will save a lot of problems in the long run. A summary of these ideas is provided in Table One. For if managers or other practitioners exhibit haste in operationalizing a MIS, the support of crucial staff persons will be lost. And because no project exists in a technical vacuum, face validity is important to the successful construction and utilization of a MIS. In short, the strictures imposed by a MIS must make sense socially.

Table 1 Summary of Key Non-technical Considerations When Developing a MIS.

1. Understand clearly the management philosophy
2. Identify key decision makers and the types of decisions that will have to be made.
3. Locate vital sources of information, and determine the most appropriate ways to gather this data.
4. Calculate the amount of effort needed to garner relevant information in a socially sensitive manner.
5. Attempt to integrate conceptual, logistical and social considerations.
6. Determine the social character of relevant data.
7. Know the culture of an organization, so that the information will flow smoothly from place to place.
8. Appreciate how the conceptual side of MIS development can enhance research and other activities.
9. Use a MIS project as an opportunity to integrate an organization

I. The first rule is quite simple: Do not attempt to resurrect an already dead information system in order to facilitate the development of a new MIS. Many managers, in the hope of increasing the speed with which a MIS can be implemented, attempt to eliminate the initial developmental stages of a system by building on a previously established, but not currently used, information system. Many times this is done to enlarge a program's data base by also using the data that are contained in this system. Yet if an information system is not currently being used, it is probably in this dormant condition for a good organizational reason. The use of an old information system, therefore, involves far more than merely reinstituting the logistical apparatus of this MIS. Also relevant should be an investigation of the programmatic problems that brought about the demise of the old system. If this type of study is not undertaken, the new MIS may be undermined by similar difficulties.

For example, the use of such data, in effect, represents secondary analysis. Little knowledge may be available pertaining to the management philosophy that was prevalent when the old MIS was inaugurated. Consequently, the goals and objectives that guided data collection will not be known. In this regard, the data processing categories present in the old system may have no utility for the new managers. Moreover, the quality of the methods adopted to gather the data present in the defunct MIS cannot be verified. Using data that may have been collected for another purpose is usually viewed as suspect. At this time the question must be addressed: What are data? Are data merely objective "things" that can be shuffled from one context to another without any loss of meaning, or are the identity and worth of information affected by situational consideration? Reliable data for a medical practitioner may be different from the knowledge deemed acceptable by workers in a welfare office (Murphy, 1979). Most important, questions related to the quality of information are not technological in scope.

II. Program evaluation develops in stages, with process assessments followed by impact studies. Impact evaluation, accordingly, is viewed typically to be the highest stage of evaluation research. As might be suspected, these two types of evaluation are based on different kinds of data. Information appropriate for process evaluation is produced during the initial stages of MIS development, while the later stages allow for the collection of the information appropriate for conducting impact research. Therefore, the growth of a MIS, similar to program evaluation, must be fostered. This means that the inaugural phases of MIS development must be used to promote the final stages of this system. Stated differently, the gradual evolution of technical factors will not necessarily guarantee the proper growth of a MIS. Much more active intervention into an organization is essential.

A variety of authors have outlined the developmental stages through which a MIS must pass (McIntyre, et. al., 1977). The initial task in information processing capability relates to identifying the natural source of the information to be collected. Next this source of data must be centrally located. Following this, the flow of information must be standardized and regulated by managerial imperatives. At this juncture a manager actually gains control of the MIS. And finally, the full capability of a MIS can be realized once specialized information requests can be handled by the system. Clearly this last stage must be reached before impact evaluation can be conducted. None of these stages should be circumvented in order to increase the speed of MIS development. For during the preliminary stages of producing a MIS is when a program's staff learn how to conceptualize the more elaborate phases of a system.

For instance, locating a data source cannot be accomplished without knowing who will use the information, the purpose for collecting it, and the management decisions that will be made. Merely increasing the presence of information technology will not insure that data flow smoothly to the proper places in an organization. Generated by technology are technical questions. Identifying the sources and uses of data, however, relate to the culture of program. These are social issues that have nothing to do with technical expertise. Accordingly, many businesses have begun to recognize that merely allowing technology to proliferate will not promote the effective use of information (Namm, 1986). The environment of an organization must be understood, before data processing will enhance the decision making of managers.

If a manager opts to skip stages, staff persons (1) will not properly relate the information collected to the services that are to be delivered, (2) will not have time to conceptualize sufficiently the data collection process, and thus (3) will not understand how the MIS fits into the overall operation of a program. Without this global perspective, the success of a MIS is placed in jeopardy. On the one hand, workers may not be motivated to promote a MIS, while, on a more technical level, the interface between management philosophy and data may be obscured. Experts say that the proper implementation of a MIS cannot be rushed, without paying a high cost with respect to personnel and technical concerns (McConkey, 1975). Basically, formulating a MIS is a conceptual exercise that should not be limited to systems design, for information must flow through social networks.

III. Ultimately a MIS should contain a historical file on each client who has been admitted to treatment. In this sense, a client can be followed throughout a particular treatment episode. In order to save time, however, many managers do not follow a coherent data collection methodology. Instead of having the data collection process based on a client's movements throughout a clinic, bits and pieces of information are provided at various points throughout treatment (Garfinkel, 1974). In management terms, data collection is situation-specific, rather than oriented by a particular case. Identical data are gathered from each client who passes through a specific in-take checkpoint in a clinic. The focus of this process is not the client, but the organization.

Obviously garnering information in this manner can cause serious problems. Such a disjointed methodology (1) does not promote information continuity, (2) does not allow for errors to be readily noted and corrected, and (3) results in a lot of "catch-up" work in terms of undertaking quality assurance checks. The major reason for these problems is that treatment continuity is not fostered, because data collection evolves around organizational requirements.

A record that is more client oriented will reduce these problems. Yet in some ways this sort of individualization is anathema to the technological imperative. Data should not be made to conform to information processing requirements, as is often the case. Additionally, the path a client follows during treatment should be viewed as the core of the organization. Data collection needs, therefore, should be based on treatment, rather than abstract organizational and technical demands. In this way, the focus of data collection can be the client, without managers feeling that they are losing control of a clinic. The point is that practitioners should not be blinded by the mystique of technology to the extent that they lose sight of the client. The collection of data must not become an end in itself. To make a MIS client-oriented, the focus of attention must be the services delivered and not data processing (Murphy and Pilotta, 1983). A data record should be built around the clients who are served.

IV. Another problem with overzealous managers is that they often confuse the management with the research system (Murphy, 1981). These systems make different demands on the data that are collected. The strength of the research system becomes apparent when variable or statistical controls are introduced into the data collection process. Yet this need for controls requires the collection of so much information on an ongoing basis that a program's staff can easily overburdened. Likewise, in order to test "crucial hypotheses" additional data must be continuously collected. As a result of the increasing pressure to collect data for research purposes, a MIS may break down. Stated simply, a research system requires more resources than a management system to be properly operationalized. A research system is used to test the null hypothesis, while a MIS is designed to collect and organize information. These different purposes should not be forgotten, or data that are useless to both systems will likely be generated.

Yet the aim of program evaluation is to conduct experiments. Is a MIS useless in this endeavor? Of course not, but a MIS must not be understood to grow into a research system following logistical refinements. Nonetheless, a MIS can prepare staff members to conduct research, if the heart of a management system is viewed to be conceptual activity. After all, conducting research requires that data be identified, variables be operationalized, and a holistic view of the phenomenon to be tested be adopted. As should be noted, all of these components of research can be part of building a MIS. If managers are skillful, the conceptual abilities that are acquired while assembling a MIS can be generalized to the research setting. This learning will not take place, however, as long as technical issues are the predominate concern of managers.

V. Planners should not initiate a MIS project without a thorough appreciation of the data to be collected, the effort that will be expended to acquire this information, and the amount of time and effort that will be needed to maintain the data base. It should be remembered that a MIS is not a neutral device, but actually imposes a conceptual scheme on data. Margaret Boden (1977) makes this point when she states that computers operate at a symbolic level and do not simply process data. How does this conceptual apparatus affect the use of a MIS? This question must not be ignored.

For example, how will the way data are understood be affected by a MIS? Are practitioners likely to avoid gathering complex information, because these data cannot be easily circumscribed? Will the quantification that usually accompanies MIS development alter how services are conceptualized and, possibly, delivered (Murphy and Pardeck, 1986). A "unit" of service may have to be defined in a way that is consistent with data processing needs, but is socially irrelevant. In other words, practitioners should recognize that maintaining a "clean" data base may come into conflict with the essential social character of information.

Additionally, those who plan to use a MIS must also remember that data cannot be simply identified, gathered, and stored. Information, in short, is supposed to be utilized. Suggested by the idea of utilization is that data will be applied. Therefore, a lot of effort is required to insure that relevant information is obtained. Yet expending too much energy in this way may unduly disrupt the operation of a program. Most important, due to the emphasis placed on relevance, social instead of technical competence is required to collect valid data. At the basis of social competence is sensitivity, rather than the principle of standardization that often underpins a MIS. Accordingly, integrating data processing requirements with the theoretical presuppositions of data and social sensitivity is vital to the viability of a MIS. Yet the contemplation needed for such a task may frustrate some managers, who are most interested in technical developments. Nonetheless, the fine balance between theoretical and logistical issues that is present in a well functioning MIS must not be disrupted.

VI. Building a MIS should not be approached as a self-contained enterprise. Instead, a MIS project should be a component of a much more expansive organizational development (OD) strategy. The opportunity should be taken, in other words, to evaluate other aspects of the organization. For example, does a program have goals and objectives? What are the nature of communication channels? How is the management philosophy that is present in an organization manifested in the everyday affairs of employees? Because a MIS has impact on practically every aspect of an organization, the opportunity is presented to study management issues that are regularly overlooked. In short, organizational assessment should be viewed as the underside of MIS development.

Specifically, in order for a MIS to operate effectively, an organization must be integrated. The key at this juncture is the idea of systematization. Contrary to traditional office practices, a MIS allows managers to extend beyond the organizational restrictions placed on space and time. Information that is gathered as part of traditional record keeping is often collected for one purpose, at a particular time, and according to a single format (Murphy, 1982). In this sense, these data collection procedures are not very flexible, in that data categories cannot be readily merged, nor can additional information be added to each collection device so that trends can be detected. Information and thus the organization remains fragmented. A MIS, on the other hand, is accompanied by a very different outlook. The strength of a MIS is that it is able to provide an integrated picture of an organization. Knowledge integration is the cornerstone of a MIS. Additionally, the planning that should accompany the implementation of a MIS can facilitate organizational cohesiveness. That is, an action plan should be formulated that is submitted to staff persons for their scrutiny. At this time, the rationale for developing a MIS should be outlined in detail. Both conceptual issues and organizational needs should be addressed. As a result of this undertaking, the members of individual departments can begin to appreciate how they fit into the overall organization. If this plan is democratically enacted, a type of organization consensus can be the result. Kurt Lewin, for instance, referred to this phenomenon as "buy in", whereby organizational boundaries begin to dissolve (Murphy, 1984). The point is that viewed as an OD issue, establishing a MIS can have organizational impact that is not limited to improved data collection.

Modern writers note correctly that technology has a mystique. The appeal of high-tech instruments is strong, because of the claim that they are rational and undaunted by human foibles. Central to this paper, however, is that managers and practitioners should not become entrapped within what Jacques Ellul (1964) calls the "technological ethic". By this he means that the lure of technology must not blind managers and practitioners to a simple fact: technology exists within a broad context comprised of values, beliefs, and commitments. And when established on these factors, instead of obscuring them, technology can improve the human condition. Yet, as suggested earlier in this paper, the success of technology is thought traditionally to be based on the separation of fact and value.

The wisdom expressed by Ellul is pertinent to installing a MIS. If a MIS is understood to exist within an organizational culture, technical considerations can be tempered by ones that are social. In this way, a lot more than improved information processing capability can be forthcoming from a MIS project. Developing a MIS can prompt thoughtful reflection about the entire operation of an organization. By looking at non-technical considerations, the human side of data collection and utilization can be enhanced. Both managers and practitioners must remember that the foundation of a MIS is not simply technology.

REFERENCES

Boden, Margaret, *Artificial Intelligence and Natural Man*. New York: Basic Books, 1977.

Ellul, Jacques, *The Technological Society*. New York: Random House, 1964.

Garfinkel, Harold, "'Good' Organizational Reasons for 'Bad' Clinical Records: In *Ethnomethodology*, edited by Roy Turner. Middlesex, England: Penguin Books, 1974, pp. 109-127.

McConkey, Dale D., *MBO For Nonprofit Organizations*. New York: AMACOM, 1975.

McIntyre, M., Attkisson, C. C. and Keller, T. W., "Components of Program Evaluation Capability in Community Mental Health Centers. In W. A. Hargreaves, C. C. Attkisson, and J. E. Sorsensen (eds). *Resource Materials For Community Mental Health Program Evaluation*. Rockville, MD: DHEW, 1977.

Murphy, John W., "Drug Program Evaluation: Outcome Measures". *Journal of Drug Education* 9 (4), 1979, pp. 309-314.

Murphy, John W., "The Management and the Research System — Is There a Difference? In *Drug Dependence and Alcoholism*, VOL II, edited by Arnold Schecter. New York: Plenum, 1981, pp. 601-608.

Murphy, John W., "Organizational Issues in Worker Ownership". *American Journal of Economics and Sociology* 43 (3), 1984, pp. 287-299.

Murphy, John W., "Some thoughts about MIS Implementation in Drug Abuse Programs", *The International Journal of the Addictions* 17(1), 1982, pp. 205-212.

Murphy, John W., and Pardeck, John T., "Technologically Mediated Therapy: A Critique". *Social Casework* 67(10), 1986, pp. 605-612.

Murphy, John W., and Pardeck, John T. "Technology in Clinical Practice and the 'Technological Ethic'", *Journal of Sociology and Social Welfare* 15(1), 1988, pp. 119-128.

Murphy, John W., Pardeck, John T., Nolden, Wesley L. and Pilotta, Joseph J. "Conceptual Issues Related to the use of Computers in Social Work Practice", *Journal of Independent Social Work*, 1(4), 1987, pp. 63-73.

Murphy, John W., and Pilotta, Joseph J., "Some Epistemological Issues Related to using the Medical Record for Organizational Decision Making". In *Qualitative Methodology, Theory and Application*, by John W. Murphy and Joseph J. Pilotta. Dubuque, IA: Kendall/Hunt, 1983, pp. 139-153.

Namm, Deborah, "The Case of the Changing Technology: Impact of Microcomputer Technology in a *Fortune* 500 Company: In *Technology and Human Productivity*, edited by John W. Murphy and John T. Pardeck. Westport, CT: Quorum Books, 1986, pp. 95-101.

13
Technological Imagery and Social Intervention

Karen A. Callaghan, PhD
Department of Sociology, Miami University

John W. Murphy, PhD
Associate Professor of Sociology, Miami University

Joseph J. Pilotta, PhD
Ohio State University

Currently technological needs-assessment strategies are being used increasingly to identify social problems. These approaches are thought to be more rigorous than those previously used, and thus are touted to generate valid data. However, planners and policy makers are mistaken when they treat technology as fundamentally a research tool, something that can greatly improve data collection. In order to understand properly modern technology, researchers must recognize that it is not simply an unbiased method that can be used at their discretion, but in fact can shape surreptitiously both the world and data, thereby giving hidden direction to a research project. A researcher's perception, in other words, is influence by technology.

As Mumford (1963) suggests, technology is a "world-view" and not just a host of neutral techniques. The central element of this viewpoint is control, in that technology aims to eliminate uncertainty, error, and inefficiency from any setting. The so-called human element is variable, while technology is not. The world, in a certain sense, is now organized in accordance to what some are calling a "technological imperative" (Wolf & Berle, 1981; Mechanic, 1982). Accordingly, technology should be introduced whenever possible, so that the human factors in any job are adequately controlled. Technological imagery, in short, has come to pervade research and policy formation. As a result, the prospects for gathering valid knowledge are believed to be enhanced, for technology is cited to be uninfluenced by situational exigencies (Ellul, 1964).

Technology deanimates the world as a result of three principles that are integral to its world-view. First, all phenomena are materialized. Everything that is known is treated as pure matter, an extended object, or, simply put, a thing to be manipulated. According to technological reason, the world consists of inanimate facts. Second, because mathematics is the language of technology, a rational calculus is adopted to outline an object's identity. Thus, only quantitative knowledge is considered reliable. Third, both the material and social world are understood to operate according to the laws of physics. In this sense, events are explained in a completely impersonal manner.

Because the technological world-view is accepted as legitimate, a key problem associated with research is overcome. That is, the impossible situation created by the introduction of dualism is resolved. Implied by the technological world-view is that facts can be differentiated from values, as well as subjectivity from objectivity. After all, the use of technology is encouraged by the belief that increased technical or procedural rigor will allow human error to be minimized. As suggested by Jean-Francois Lyotard (1984), technology serves as a sort of "prosthetic aid". In other words, human perception can be reinforced by devices that are allegedly value-free. Through the increased use of research technology, intervention can be guided by "trained perception." As a result of transforming judgments into technical operations, the illusion can be perpetrated that all values are purged from research. Indeed, most persons tend to believe that methodological axioms are unbiased. By clearly operationalizing every procedure, interpretation is assumed to be moved to the periphery of the data collection process. Therefore, the focus of research becomes technical competence. The mastery of technique is thought to lead to the discovery of valid knowledge, because following standardized instructions is not believed to involve interpretation.

Hence the procurement of information is neutralized. Research instruments are transformed into implements for harvesting data. Objective facts are identified, garnered, and classified. Accuracy comes to be equated with precision. Moreover, questions of health and illness are no longer important, but rather a structurally defined normative standard is the focus attention. Instead of judged as relevant or irrelevant, data are compared to this standard. And intervention is inaugurated when deviation from this norm is too great. In short, due to technological imagery research is undertaken in a very mechanistic manner.

THE METHODOLOGICAL IMPORTANCE OF TECHNOLOGICAL IMAGERY

Clearly the technological world-view affects the study of social life. This occurs because the following facets of social existence are defined in technological terms: (1) the structure of order, (2) the characteristics of data, (3) the rationale for behavior, and (4) the laws of society. As might be expected, this world-view construes society in such a manner that technological methodologies are deemed most appropriate for conducting social research. Although this point will be expatiated upon later, most important at this juncture is how technological rationality misconstrues social "reality."

1. When conceived technologically, order is depicted in a manner consistent with ontological realism. As Stark (1963, pp. 1-13) points out, realists believe that society has an existence of its own, divorced from its members. Society is an objective thing, or a reality *sui generis*, as labeled by Durkheim. Such a dualistic portrayal of society is certainly technological, since order is presented as a spatial entity. Sometimes, as in the work of Talcott Parsons, society is referred to as a system, thereby invoking imagery that is consistent with technological rationality. Specifically, when understood as a system, society is envisioned to be a self-contained, well-integrated machine, which is able to control individuals and secure order. As an objective entity, society can supply a base for norms that is uncontaminated by the capriciousness associated with individuals.

2. Since society is thought to be a "thing", data are assumed to be objective. In the classic sense, society has an identity that is not influenced by human action. Clearly this is consistent with the idea that societal norms are sustained by a source that is immune to individual interpretation. Accordingly, social phenomena are believed to have objective traits that are readily visible to the trained observer. The aim of research, stated simply, is to document these social indices, so that a society's problems, for example, are accurately revealed. In order to gain access to facts, however, researchers must overcome the element of interpretation and address obtrusive events. Hence, the research act must be neutralized, for truth is equated with objectivity.

3. When society is construed dualistically, individuals usually are treated as the source of subjectivity. According to Foucault, this style of Cartesianism suggests that individuals are devoid of rationality, since subjectivity is basically whimsical. As a consequence of this negative view of subjectivity, individuals are assumed to lack self-direction, because irrationality, by definition, does not have an orientation. Yet this poses a problem: How is behavior initiated? The answer that is typically given is that persons are *caused* to act by objective social factors. In this sense, social structure acts as a catalyst that motivates a person to pursue a particular course of action. Traditionally it is thought that insight is gained into behavior by studying these objective social conditions.

4. Society is considered the entity that shapes individuals. Moreover, the impact that social forces exert when influencing behavior is not thought to be altered by individual interpretation. Thus, social laws are not contingent upon, or subject to, existential exigencies, but are similar to those which underpin the physical world. These laws specify the relationships between structural conditions and behavior,

and understanding an individual's actions is thought to be related directly to the extent to which these causal links have been tested and documented.

In sum, the technological world-view describes society in functional terms. That is, society is viewed as being greater than the sum of its parts, while these components are regulated by the rules which legitimize the social system. An individual's identity is thus structurally determined, as his or her behavior is specified by social roles. Consequently, researchers focus their attention on the social system. The human element, accordingly, is diminished in importance when conducting social research.

For example, coincident with functionalist social imagery is the belief that the family is a microcosm of the larger society. Additionally, the family is conceptualized as a system having an identity different from its parts. Rational behavior, moreover, is evaluated on the basis of how much a person contributes to maintaining a family's equilibrium. As with functionalist theory in general, an externalized locus of normative control is offered, along with a structural definition of legitimate behavior. Facts about family life are identified in systemic terms, while all problems are posed as structural issues.

Technological Imagery and the Assessment of Needs

The purpose of a needs assessment is to gather information about the number of persons who might require the services of a specific agency. Stated otherwise, the aim is to discover who is "at risk", for instance, of becoming a drug or alcohol abuser, a delinquent, or a psychiatric patient. In order to make such a determination, data must be collected pertaining to the kinds of persons who reside in a community, in addition to environmental conditions. Subsequently, it is possible to predict the number and types of persons who might seek treatment. This strategy is considered essential for properly implementing both preventive and corrective policies. Without an assessment of need, how can services be delivered in an effective and efficient manner?

Accompanying the recent proliferation of technology has been an increase in technological needs-assessment procedures. Because these procedures are standardized, they are thought to produce high-quality data. Information on social life is procured in the following way: First, data are identified and selected in terms of their empirical properties. Data, simply put, are objectified. Second, because empirical indicators are not ambiguous, they can be systematically formalized. As might be expected, this is accomplished by giving phenomena a quantitative, or numerical, identity. Third, the social significance of data is extrapolated from their surface qualities. Thus individuals are treated as "black boxes", who merely respond to objective events. In this way, human variability is controlled. When social policies are predicated upon such evidence, a causal link is assumed to exist between empirical data and behavior. And fourth, surface data are presumed to be indicative of underlying social laws, on which policies are supposed to be based.

These burgeoning needs-assessment strategies are mostly analytical techniques, which rely heavily on computer models. Data are selected and prepared in a manner that is consistent with the logistical demands of computerization. In many respects, the language of computerization determines the image of a community, since all information must conform to the specifications imposed by data processing. Data must be organized so that they are compatible with computer logic, which may distort their social significance. Nonetheless, the most popular methods for conducting technological needs assessments utilize simulations, Bayesian decision-making logic, cost-effectiveness algorithms, actuarial tables, forecasting models, and social indicator analysis to generate and assess data.

These procedures are cited as having the following benefits. First, they are quick and easy to perform, in that most of the data are already available in clients' records, census reports, and document filed by city planners Second, because of this availability of data, technological needs assessments are cheaper to conduct than, for example, surveys or interviews. Third, data are uniform because they are produced in a standardized manner. Fourth, this results in increased precision, since judgments are minimized. And fifth, findings are believed to be reliable because they reflect this methodological rigor. In general, technological needs assessments are deemed desirable because they are assumed to be thoroughly rational and, thus, scientific, as the following examples illustrate. Most important at this juncture is that technologically-based practices are believed to be valid, because particular assumptions about reality are accepted.

Garbarino (1980) contends that the best method of predicting child abuse is to identify "high-risk neighborhoods". This shifts the emphases from the individual to the social nature of the problem. However, the factors used to define "neighborhood" impose limitations. Specifically, a neighborhood is associated with a few objective indices, such as socioeconomic status, quality of housing, employment, and geographic area (Garbarino & Gilliam, 1980; Volpe, Breton, & Mitton, 1980; Straus, Gelles, & Steinmetz, 1981). Community psychologists state that these variables constitute the cornerstone of the "ecological model" (Mann, 1978, pp. 185-227). Social workers and researchers who adopt this approach argue that neighborhoods should be screened regularly, since those with high unemployment, transience, and substandard housing also are likely to have a high rate of child abuse.

Tierney and Corwin (1983) propose a similar strategy for studying the prevalence of child sexual abuse, although they refer to it as a "systems approach". As with the ecological model, systems analysis assesses a problem in a holistic manner. In this particular case, the key variables studied are socioeconomic status, family structure, psychological traits, and precipitating events. However, these elements are operationalized solely in empirical terms, as if they are phenomena which persons encounter and never question.

Both the ecological and systems models conceive a person's environment as a force that *causes* behavior. It is believed that undesirable conditions can weaken a person's adaptive abilities and produce violent behavior. By accurately identifying these important environmental determinants, planners can focus their intervention activities and prevent family violence. In each case, data are formalized in such a way that they can be utilized in a computer simulation of community life. On the basis of the number of indices present in an area, in addition to how they are combined, probability statements can be made about the likelihood of child abuse occurring.

A variety of strategies have been used to predict drug abuse. For example, Leon Hunt analysis, a forecasting technique, is one of the most popular methods for calculating the prevalence of heroin use in a community (Hunt, 1974). This procedure is based on the idea that a certain percentage of the heroin addicts in a population enter treatment during any one year. By counting the heroin users who enter treatment during the first year, the Leon Hunt method projects the number of addicts in the community and the rate at which they will seek treatment during each of the following four years. Planners like this methodology because it not only provides an estimate of the prevalence of addicts, but when they can be expected to solicit professional help. Along this line, planners also regularly use both linear and nonlinear models to predict future program intakes on the basis of prior treatment rates.

Drug abuse planners also consult a variety of social indicators when conducting needs assessments (Lavenhar, 1980). For example, the frequency of overdose deaths is thought to be related to the size of the addict population. The arrest patterns of heroin addicts also is used as an index of the number of users in a community. Additionally, fluctuations in drug purity are assumed to be related to program utilization: as drug purity decreases, more addicts are expected to enroll in treatment programs.

One further example relates to how mental health services are planned. Although the 1963 Community Mental Health Center Act mandated the use of community-based planning, recent research suggests that planners overwhelmingly employ measures of illness that are insensitive to a community's problems (Pilotta, Murphy, Jones, & Wilson, 1983). Specifically, they often use census data to describe the type of housing, rate of transience, and level of education in a community. These data are organized into an actuarial table, thereby enabling predictions to be made about the rate and types of illness in that location. Seldom are community members contacted directly in order to assess their needs. Need, instead, is defined in statistical terms.

These needs-assessment strategies are referred to jokingly by many planners as "quick and dirty", although theoretically they are supposed to produce high-quality data. But because funding for social service programs is often subject to reduction, research, which is given a low priority, is often undertaken in the most inexpensive manner possible. Yet these technological methods may eventually prove to be very costly. For they may result in the formulation of irrelevant, insensitive, and possibly disruptive social policies. Because data are not gathered in a socially sensitive manner, erroneous information may be produced by policy research. Contrary to the view of many policy makers, community-based research may actually save money over the long run because this approach to studying social life does not evolve around technical issues.

A Community's Self-Perception and the Nature of Social Reality

Most problematic about technological needs assessments is that they are asocial. Specifically, interpretation is ignored, and thus social reality is easily misconstrued. A social problem, therefore, is associated with particular biological, psychological, or sociological traits. Those who use technological methodologies believe that social intervention can be initiated on the basis of information relevant to these traits. Once the facts related to a problem have been identified, remedial action can be properly focused. When based on empirical evidence, the proposals advanced by planners are given more credence.

Community-based researchers, on the other hand, maintain that such an insensitive approach to conceptualizing knowledge will not necessarily result in appropriate and timely treatment (Murphy & Pilotta, 1983a, 1983b). They argue that a social problem has a "career", which must be known if a malady is to be understood, cured, or prevented. Using Matza's (1964) imagery, persons "drift" in and out of being "at risk", a condition that is not merely associated with obtrusive characteristics. Therefore, conducting a needs assessment becomes slightly more complex, since the social nature of a problem cannot be ignored, as with technologically substantiated research. Community-oriented researchers view social reality as follows.

1. All behavior is mediated by human action: persons define themselves and their environment. Hence, behavioral norms cannot necessarily be assessed according to their empirical qualities. So-called facts have meaning that must be understood, before they can be classified. Before any intervention is initiated, planners must take care to ensure that community members view the behavior that is to be preempted as problematic. In this sense, policy makers must be sensitive to the symbolic meaning of behavior. Health or illness is not necessarily a medical phenomenon, but something that is socially determined.

2. A problem is not static but related to crisis episodes. These episodes, moreover, are not part of an evolutionary or developmental path that all persons must traverse. Instead, these crises are intimately intertwined with human biography, and therefore their parameters have an existential character. Hence effort should be devoted to learning how persons explain illness, cope with this problem, and interact with their friends and neighbors when they are sick. Crisis episodes are managed by persons redefining their reality.

3. Persons are not immediately identified as sick following the appearance of symptoms. Rather, communities have a repertoire of coping strategies designed to keep the effects of disruptive behavior to a minimum (Scheff, 1966). Only when these coping mechanisms break down does deviant behavior become problematic. By documenting these coping strategies, planners can know how, when, and why they fail, thus revealing the factors that would make intervention most propitious. Most important, the rationality that underpins these coping mechanisms may appear to be irrational. Nonetheless, every definition of reality is based on assumptions that make sense, if their situational relevance is understood. A proper intervention can occur only when the interpretive "world" of a client is appreciated.

4. Those requiring assistance usually do not seek professional help first. Numerous community resources are utilized before outside treatment is sought (Mechanic, 1980). Information should be obtained about these local networks, for they are instrumental in keeping a problem "hidden" from authorities. Obviously, information pertaining to a community's networks can assist planners in pinpointing when and where intervention should be initiated. Nonetheless, these networks are not necessarily associated with ecological boundaries. A community, rather, should be treated as a domain persons define as important. The commitment exhibited by persons to a location establishes the parameters of a community.

5. Not only do community networks influence help-seeking behavior, they also may provide the only available means of providing information and treatment. Unless a planner is aware of the key persons and institutions that unite a community, treatment and prevention become haphazard. Thus treatment and prevention should not be based solely on the technical competence of planners. More important, planners must achieve a level of social competence which allows them to comprehend the existential fabric of a community. Without this insight, intervention programs may never reach the persons they are designed to assist.

Conclusion

Recent federal budget cuts have increased the appeal of technological needs-assessment methods. These techniques can be implemented cheaply and quickly, and enable planners to meet minimum evaluation requirements. Unfortunately, because of the imagery that accompanies the used of technology-based methodologies, the human element is purged from these procedures. As a result, social phenomena are conceptualized abstractly, for the role played by human interpretation in shaping the environment is eviscerated. Facts are collected that are devoid of social meaning.

Without an understanding of the social significance of behavior, it is difficult to plan intervention programs. A problem does not exist in a vacuum but within a matrix of interpersonal relations, and thus can be analyzed properly only if its social context is appreciated. Because technological research strategies obscure the social side of human action, they must be viewed as generating data of limited value. In order to increase both the reliability and validity of data, policy research must reveal the human core of society. This requires researchers to supplement their technical competence with social sensitivity.

A socially sensitive needs assessment should not be value-free, but value-based. The values that sustain a community's judgments must be assessed, before a particular behavior can be properly classified. Without this sort of insight, technically correct but socially inappropriate policies may be implemented. Certainly, such insensitivity is not therapeutic. Yet obscured by the imagery of technology are the values that sustain the reality persons accept as real.

REFERENCES

Bell, D. (1978). *The cultural contradictions of capitalism.* New York: Basic Books.

Berger, P. L., Berger, B., & Kellner, H. (1973). *The homeless mind.* New York: Random House.

Ellul, J. (1964). *The technological society.* New York: Random House.

Garbarino, J. (1980). Preventing child maltreatment. In R. H. Price, R. F. Ketterer, B. C. Bader, & J. Monahan (Eds.), *Prevention in mental health* (pp. 63-79). Beverly Hills, CA: Sage.

Garbarino, H., & Gilliam, G. (1980). *Understanding abusive families.* Lexington, MA: D.C. Heath and Co..

Hunt, L. G. (1974). *Recent spread of heroin use in the United States: Unanswered questions.* Washington, DC: Drug Abuse Council.

Lavenhar, M. A. (1980). Methodology in community research. In S. Einstein (Ed.), *The community's response to drug use* (pp.245-304). New York: Pergamon Press.

Mann, P. A. (1978). *Community psychology.* New York: Macmillan.

Matza, D. (1980). *Mental health and social policy.* Englewood Cliffs, NJ: Prentice-Hall.

Mechanic, D. (1982). The growth of medical technology: Implications for medical care. In J. B. McKinlay (Ed.), *Technology and the future of health care* (pp. 1-18). Cambridge, MA: MIT Press.

Mumford, L. (1963). *Technics and civilization.* New York: Harcourt, Brace, and World.

Murphy, J. W., & Pilotta, J. J. (Ed.). (1983a). *Qualitative methodology, theory and application: A guide for the social practitioner.* Dubuque, IA: Kendall/Hunt.

Murphy, J. W., & Pilotta, J. J. (1983b). Community-based evaluation for criminal justice planning. *Social Service Review*, 57(3), 465-476

Pilotta, J. J., Murphy, J. W., Jones, T., Wilson, E. (1983). Research note: Trends in community perception of social service planning. *Evaluation and the Health Professions*, 6(1), 131-135.

Scheff, T. J. (1966). *Being mentally ill.* Chicago: Aldine.

Stark, W. (1963). *The fundamental forms of social thought.* New York: Fordham University Press.

Straus, M. A., Gelles, R. J., Steinmetz, S. K. (1981). *Behind closed doors.* Garden City, NY: Doubleday.

Tierney, K. J., & Corwin, D. L. (1983). Exploring intrafamilial child sexual abuse. In D. Finkelhor, R.J., Gelles, G. T. Hotaling, & M. A. Straus (Ed.), *The dark side of families: Current family violence research* (pp. 102-116). Beverly Hills, CA:Sage.

Volpe, R., Breton, M., & Mitton, J. (1980). *The maltreatment of the school-aged child.* Lexington, MA: D. C. Heath and Company.

Wolf, S., & Berle, B. B. (Ed.). (1981). *The technological imperative in medicine.* New York: Plenum.

Index